THE
LAUNDRY LIST

The ACoA
(Adult Children of Alcoholics)
Experience

By the co-founder of ACoA
and originator of The Laundry List

TONY A.
with DAN F.

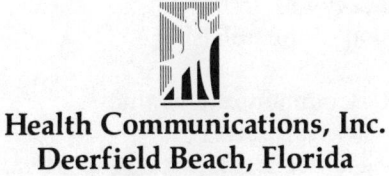

Health Communications, Inc.
Deerfield Beach, Florida

©1991 Tony A. with Dan F.
ISBN 1-55874-105-4

Publisher: Health Communications, Inc.
            3201 S.W. 15th Street
            Deerfield Beach, Florida 33442-8190

DEDICATION

To My Higher Power
and
My Wife Carline

ACKNOWLEDGMENTS

To Dan F., my dear friend and partner in the ACoA Experience.

To Cindy, who invited me to my first ACoA Meeting.

To Chris F., who typed the *Problem-Solution* the day I wrote it and made the *solution* sound better.

To Barry, who when I read the *Problem-Solution* for the first time at St. Jean Baptist's Church in New York City, said, "That's my Laundry List."

To Jerry Rathburn, whose perseverance in finding the author of the Laundry List helped make this book a reality.

To Bill W. and Dr. Bob, the founders of Alcoholics Anonymous. Without the 12 Steps of AA, the ACoA movement would not have been started.

To Lois W., the founder of Al-Anon, where the first ACoA group got together.

To Alateen because it was a small group of Alateen graduates that first formed ACoA.

And to Cynthia, my daughter who directed me toward the spiritual path when she was only a child; to John, my son who joined me in meditation and the spiritual path; to Lark, my daughter whose love of animals and concern for planet earth has always inspired me and to Mowry, my two-year-old daughter who will be the first of my children not to be brought up in an alcoholic home. May I be a better father than I was before.

And to Joe Varney, who has influenced me to become a better person; to Tom Duane, whose love, kindness and humor has made my life richer; to my stepson, Mike — I love him. To John

Miller, the kindest man I have ever known; to John J. Ryan III —
my brother; to Carl, Helen and Charlie. Thank you for your
love; to my dear sister P. and her husband L. whose love and
support have always been with me; to Fagie M. — a true lady
and dear friend; to Adrian A., a gentle and lovely soul. To Peter
Glasheen who suggested that Dan F. and I write this book
together; to Bob Cole, one of the brightest men I ever met; to
Jim Robinson, a dear friend and spiritual companion; to Wilma
Coates, my loving spiritual teacher who taught me the principles of the Infinite Way and introduced me to the works of Joel
Goldsmith and Gopi Krishna.

To Peter Vegso and Gary Seidler of Health Communications,
who by publishing books for Adult Children have acknowledged our problems, given us support and offered us positive
help for recovery. With their books they have helped hundreds
of thousands of people. We thank you both! We appreciate you!

And to Andrew Meacham whose wonderful ability as a wri-
ter came through in his article about me in *Changes Magazine*. I
thank him for the kindness and understanding he gave me. To
my editors, Marie Stilkind and Naomi Lucks, whose patience
and editing skills have been invaluable. And to all the produc-
tion, press and shipping staff at Health Communications, I thank
you. Without you, this book would not exist.

Tony A.

CONTENTS

Foreword:
A Physician's Perspective

To paraphrase an old cliche, "Once I didn't know what an ACoA was, and now I find out I am one."

The powerful healing movement of adult children of alcoholics (ACoA) as pioneered by Tony A. is helping thousands of people around the world each day. I am one of those people.

I met Tony in 1982 at the first ACoA meeting I attended. He was leading the group and had just begun to read the Laundry List when I entered. I had some very strong mixed emotions. The list hit me right between the eyes, but at the same time I felt sorry for what I termed this "group of lost souls" who had been so greatly abused as children. Sure, I could identify with them, but my case wasn't nearly so severe. I breathed a little easier after this observation.

My "mistake," if you will, was that I followed their suggestion and kept coming back to meetings. Inevitably "them" became "us." As I attended meetings my smugness disappeared and wretching feelings almost turned me inside out. There was serious and hard work for me to do here, but there were also promises of great rewards if I stuck to the program.

How could a person with such advantages and so many successes feel so confused and erratic inside? For me, this had always been a great unsolvable mystery. Slowly, however, what my life was really about began to be revealed to me.

I was raised by a mother who was suffering from alcoholism. I gradually began to understand that our whole family was suffering with alcoholism, even though the only one who drank alcohol heavily was my mother.

As I grew toward adulthood, I mostly repressed memories of what a lonely lost child I was. In high school I found what I thought was the secret to happiness — success in academics and, later on, in my profession. I graduated from high school at age 16, college at age 19 — Phi Beta Kappa — and medical school at age 23. A few years later I finished my residency in psychiatry but retained a kind of preoccupation with helping alcoholics — my own mother being number one on my list of people I wanted to see recover.

My professional life had a long series of pioneering achievements. I established the first ongoing inpatient service for alcoholics in any branch of the U.S. military. I directed two state alcohol and drug programs, wrote an internationally accepted textbook on alcoholism and established the first private inpatient service for alcohol and drug treatment in Florida. The same year I established the first inpatient program for families of alcoholics anywhere in the world. I was dedicated to my profession and was very successful. I loved my wife and three sons.

Despite all this my life began to unravel. I was a workaholic and my marriage and family began to fall apart. I was depressed and finally suicidal and desperate.

I remained, figuring I must have got the wrong partner the first time. Divorce proved me wrong again. I changed homes, changed friends, changed places where I worked, and even took several years of leave from my profession. But inside and outside the turmoil continued. What happened to the magic key to life I thought I had? Where was the happiness all of my successes were supposed to give me?

Then I began to hear and understand the message of ACoA. I had made success and people my gods, but they were false gods.

The 12-Step slogan, "It works if you work it" was quite accurate. As I practiced the ACoA principles of recovery and other spiritually based activities (Co-dependency anonymous, daily prayer and meditation, and commitment to active participation in a faith of my choice), the promises of recovery began to bloom for me.

The fruits of my recovery have been of two kinds, personal and professional. I have developed a new, very committed relationship with a spiritual being, my Higher Power and God of my understanding, which became the number one priority in my life. I no longer define happiness in material terms such as professional achievements or money; and I value people highly but they were no longer my gods. Instead I redefined happiness and success as becoming the best human being I could be — more caring, more sensitive and responsible, more open in revealing who I really am and more interested in who others really are.

As a result of these internal changes, my relationships with my family and other people became more caring and relaxed. I no longer had a need to try to control all those people whom I never really controlled anyway. I began experiencing serenity for the first time in my life. Now I truly like myself. I practice forgiveness in my daily affairs. This was truly a spiritual awakening.

The other major group of blessings center on my professional career in the field of chemical dependency. My ability to understand patients and dysfunctional families increased dramatically. I took leadership in making ACoA issues and principles of recovery a basic component of the intense inpatient chemical dependency treatment center in which I was involved.

The pebbles that Tony A. and Dan F. have dropped into the pond of recovery by writing this book will, I believe, create ripples in far distant places. The lessons contained in this book have changed my life dramatically for the better, and they have improved the lives of countless others who work the program. We all owe a debt of gratitude to them for helping make our search for serenity a more understandable journey.

Ronald J. Catanzaro, M.D.
Palm Beach Institute

Introduction

Recent government statistics indicate that more than 30 million Americans have alcoholic parents. This is a staggering figure. Even more important is the fact that many millions, perhaps most of them, are not aware of the fact that alcoholism is a family disease that affects all members of the household.

Children who live in an alcoholic environment tend to take on many of the characteristics of the family illness. Men and women who grew up in an alcoholic household suffer from a broad spectrum of difficulties, including chronic anxiety, depression, extreme fear of rejection, inability to express feelings, rigidity of personality and destructively low self-esteem. No family member escapes without some damaging emotional scars. Although children of alcoholics may vow never to be like their drunken parents, and go to great lengths to distance themselves from the family through a better education and different lifestyle, much of the emotional content of the disease stays with them until they enter recovery.

ACoA—Adult Children of Alcoholics—is a worldwide recovery program. It is available to all who have suffered the pain and anguish of being raised in an alcoholic home. The ACoA recovery program is a fellowship that speaks directly to the problems experienced by men and women brought up in a family crippled by alcoholism. Our purpose in writing this book is to present this recovery program to you, to share with you what we have learned from thousands of members and to help you realize a happier, richer life, free of limiting defenses and destructive behavior. This book is a primer and guide that can help you understand the nature of the ACoA program, how it works, the many issues that confront recovering ACoAs and the practical steps involved in achieving a successful recovery.

The tools of recovery and discovery described in this book were developed over the first 12 years of the program's existence. They work—but only if the individual member is willing to *do* the work. Recovery is a complex process. We cannot return to childhood and ask our parents to love us in the way that we needed to be loved. It just can't be done. As ACoAs we need to learn how to nurture and fulfill ourselves. We need to look within, find the origins of our feelings and come to understand our difficulties and the role we play in causing them.

This is all possible within the framework of the ACoA program. Those of us who have lived through the nightmare of family alcoholism need a safe and secure environment where we can unburden ourselves, be brought closer to our painful childhood feelings and learn that we are not alone in our struggle. As ACóAs we have paid a tremendous price to reach this point of recovery.

The recovery process works. You don't have to accept your life the way that it is now. You can change. The ACoA recovery program has produced many miracles: I have seen many of them and I am one of them. In ACoA members learn about the critically important elements of the recovery process, including the resistance and denial and how they operate to limit growth. All of these subjects are comprehensively covered in this book.

Over the years I have personally observed the recovery efforts of literally thousands of ACoAs. We have shared our pain and grief, success and setbacks. Out of this continuing exchange I have come to see more clearly the patterns of behavior that frustrate growth, the unrealistic expectations, the limited grasp of the recovery process. In this book I have tried to address these difficulties in a meaningful way.

A principal mission of the ACoA recovery program is to help members gain some clarity about their personal relationships, family ties, work, personal goals and other key issues. Throughout the book I have concentrated on the healing power of group support, the sharing of long-buried family secrets, the experiencing of painful childhood feelings and the willingness to consider a spiritual path. Much of the emphasis is on action and the need to turn inward and develop an understanding of who we became and how this can be changed.

Most of all this book is about hope. The first ACoA group ever formed took as a name for itself "Hope For Adult Children Of Alcoholics." Today's ACoA program continues to offer that hope to each and every adult child of an alcoholic who is willing to take that first step toward recovery.

Tony A.

The Original Laundry List

1. We became isolated and afraid of people and authority figures.
2. We became approval seekers and lost our identity in the process.
3. We are frightened by angry people and any personal criticism.
4. We either become alcoholics, marry them or both, or find another compulsive personality such as a workaholic to fulfill our sick abandonment needs.
5. We live life from the viewpoint of victims and are attracted by that weakness in our love and friendship relationships.
6. We have an overdeveloped sense of responsibility and it is easier for us to be concerned with others rather than ourselves; this enables us not to look too closely at our own faults, etc.
7. We get guilt feelings when we stand up for ourselves instead of giving in to others.
8. We became addicted to excitement.
9. We confuse love and pity and tend to "love" people we can "pity" and "rescue."
10. We have "stuffed" our feelings from our traumatic childhoods and have lost the ability to feel or express our feelings because it hurts so much (Denial).
11. We judge ourselves harshly and have a very low sense of self-esteem.
12. We are dependent personalities who are terrified of abandonment and will do anything to hold on to a relationship in order *not* to experience painful abandonment feelings, which we received from living with sick people who were never there emotionally for us.
13. Alcoholism is a family disease; and we became para-alcoholics and took on the characteristics of that disease even though we did not pick up the drink.
14. Para-alcoholics are reactors rather than actors.

The ACoA
12 Steps Of Recovery

1. We admitted that we were powerless over the effects of living with alcoholism and that our lives had become unmanageable.

2. We came to believe that a power greater than ourselves could bring us clarity.

3. We made a decision to practice self-love and to trust in a Higher Power of our understanding.

4. We made a searching and blameless inventory of our parents because, in essence, we had become them.

5. We admitted to our Higher Power, to ourselves and to another human being the exact nature of our childhood abandonment.

6. We were entirely ready to begin the healing process with the aid of our Higher Power.

7. We humbly asked our Higher Power to help us with our healing process.

8. We became willing to open ourselves to receive the unconditional love of our Higher Power.

9. We became willing to accept our own unconditional love by understanding that our Higher Power loves us unconditionally.

10. We continued to take personal inventory and to love and approve of ourselves.

11. We sought through prayer and meditation to improve our conscious contact with our Higher Power, praying only for knowledge of its will for us and the power to carry it out.

12. We have had a spiritual awakening as a result of taking these steps, and we continue to love ourselves and to practice these principles in all our affairs.

Who Is Tony A.?

I was born on November 4, 1927, and raised in New York City. My mother was a Christian and my father was a Jew, and I was brought up as an Episcopalian. Both of my parents were alcoholics.

My father was a successful stockbroker on Wall Street, so we were well provided for materially. Emotionally, however, our family was impoverished. From the beginning my life was touched by the insanity of an alcoholic household.

One evening, when I was one year old, my parents went out to dinner. It was the servants' night off and they left me in the care of my 19-year-old uncle, an alcoholic whom my father was trying to help out of a tight spot. When my parents returned from their night out, they discovered his body in my bedroom, a gun and a bottle of booze at his side. He had shot himself in the head, in an alcoholic stupor, and my crib was splattered with his blood and brains. From that time on loud noises always terrified me.

Soon after my uncle's suicide, my parents had a trial separation — because of her drinking, my father said. He went off to Hawaii, and my mother led a single life of Prohibition parties and drinking in a world peopled by wealthy underworld figures.

1

One night she went to a party at the Savoy Plaza and never returned home. She was found dead, her pearl necklace wrapped tightly around her neck. She was 26 years old. Whether she had been murdered or had simply passed out after a night of drinking and been accidentally asphyxiated, no one ever discovered.

My mother's death had a devastating impact on my life. I was barely two years old, yet I can still remember lying in my crib crying, "I want my mummy. I want my mummy," and wondering what I had done that was so bad that she wouldn't come back to me. My stomach ached for days. To this day I get terrible pains in my stomach whenever I experience grief, loss or abandonment.

My father remarried within a year and my stepmother soon became enmeshed in the dynamics of my father's alcoholism. When my father was drinking, he would sometimes become cruel. I can recall vividly his brutal reaction to a typical childhood incident.

My father came home one evening and discovered that I had failed to lift the toilet seat when I had to urinate, and had accidentally wet the toilet seat. He came storming into my bedroom, where my nurse was reading me a bedtime story. She screamed at him to stop as he snatched me up and dragged me into the bathroom. In a rage he rubbed my face around the rim of the toilet seat — the same way he trained our dog when he made a mistake. I was literally shaking after this punishment. The next morning when I went into his room to apologize, I found that he seemed to have no recollection of the incident.

I thought I must have done something too awful to be discussed. I was not old enough to know that in my home the punishment was always out of proportion to the crime. Emotionally I felt that my father had abandoned me. I could no longer trust him to care for me. I felt hurt and guilty and very much alone. The experience left me fearful of him and all authority figures.

My father never punished me physically again after this incident, save for a few slaps in the face when he was annoyed with my behavior. Fortunately those times were few. To avoid his wrath I became a model son, always obedient and alert.

My stepmother was a very complex woman with problems of her own. She struggled with dependency on alcohol, sleeping pills and diet pills for years.

She was generally supportive and concerned about me, but sometimes I got very mixed signals.

Like my father, she verbally abused me, attacking me bitterly. On occasion she was physically abusive. When enraged, she would stare at me angrily and force me to look into her eyes. I am still uncomfortable around angry abusive women and have trouble confronting them.

For years my father would take me to visit my grandmother in her suite at the Waldorf Astoria every Sunday, after which we would have a dinner I was too upset to eat. These visits were a torture and an embarrassment. She would spend the entire visit criticizing and berating my father, screaming that he was a rotten failure as a son and constantly recounting his faults. I felt guilt and shame over the whole thing whenever she turned her attention toward me. After all, I was my father's son. If he was no good, how then was I?

When I was ten, my grandmother became depressed and committed suicide by swimming out to sea. I felt great relief when I heard she had died, principally because I was spared any more Sunday visits.

Shortly after her death I began to feel guilty about my relief at not having to visit her anymore. What kind of dutiful grandson would have such sick selfish thoughts? I felt no sadness or loss, just relief followed by guilt.

In 1939, when Hitler was killing Jews in Germany, I found a note in my school desk that was to change my life. The note said, "Tony is a dirty Jew." I felt shame and embarrassment and fear. All I could do was stare down at my desk. Stunned and shaken, I showed the note to my father, who responded by telling me that I was only half-Jewish. I felt shocked by his reply, which I took to mean that I was only "half-dirty."

Soon thereafter my father became very troubled about anti-Semitism in this country and decided to change the family name. I suggested the name of my favorite chemistry teacher, and it became our new legal name.

The following year I was sent away to boarding school in Virginia, where no one would know about my name change. My best friend also attended this school with me. My father paid his tuition so I would not be lonely. By now, however, concealment and secrecy about my family origins was a way of life. Clearly I was unacceptable as a half-Jew. I was being taught to deny my family heritage—or at least one-half of it.

At boarding school I escaped the oppressive atmosphere of my family's alcoholism but replaced it with worry that my closest friend would reveal my dark secret. It got so I couldn't sleep at night and the school nurse began giving me sleeping pills. This was marvelous! I had a substance that quickly helped me overcome my worry and concern. As a way to change feelings, I see it now as the beginning of my addictive behavior.

The anti-Semitism issue had a profound effect on me. I became overly sensitive to what other people thought of me. I tried to please everyone, but couldn't trust anyone. Worst of all, I did not accept myself. I felt flawed and inferior and that there was something very wrong with me.

I had been sent away to boarding school to hide, and at first I did miserably. But after two years I transferred to another school. There I was number one on the tennis team, ran the class newspaper and became editor of the yearbook — all in an effort to be accepted.

After graduation I moved on to the University of Virginia, where I joined a Christian fraternity. Mindful of my father's injunction — "If you ever reveal that you are half-Jewish, I will disown you" — I told everyone that I was 100 percent Christian, a condition for fraternity membership. I was in a terrible bind and it forced me to live a lie. Once again my father had abandoned me. I felt lost and alone in my deception.

At the University I played tennis, shot pool and gambled. I didn't touch liquor — my father and I had made a pact that he would give me a sizable sum of money if I refrained from any alcohol until I was 21 years old. As a substitute I selected gambling—mostly poker, and shooting craps.

When I was at boarding school and college, my father began acting out in strange ways. He was heavily in the grips of alcoholism. His behavior became more bizarre and my stepmother began taking him to mental health clinics. She soon became worn out with this and turned the task over to me.

I remember leaving him at the different facilities, always feeling guilty that I was leaving him there alone and so forlorn. Even though he had asked me to bring him there, he would invariably say to me, "How can you leave me in a place like this?" I felt sad that my father was in such a desperate way and needed to go to such places. It was a depressing scene. I had ample material comforts but little in the way of stability or nurturing by my parents. It was all very confusing and frightening.

All of these events made me feel different and apart. I was always fearful that those I was with would discover my name change. Concealment and acceptance became primary themes in my relationships with others. Behind it all was a lot of self-loathing and very little self-acceptance.

When I graduated from college, I returned to New York and became a stockbroker, following in my father's footsteps. One major difference, however, was the way in which I chose to present myself. For so long I had hidden my Jewish heritage and hated my past. Now I became vocal regarding my Jewish/Christian roots. In fact I jammed it down people's throats, testing their reactions. That way, if someone became my friend, at least I knew he or she was aware that I was part Jewish and accepted me as I was. I was truly sensitized to this issue and it deeply distorted my thoughts and actions. I put people through difficult tests to assure myself that they were real friends.

With women I learned to be a consummate people-pleaser, manipulator and abandoner. My goal was to avoid the terror I felt if they displayed any anger, or the guilt I felt when I left them. "Keep them happy, distracted and satisfied and they won't abandon me."

As a result of my childhood experiences the early days in ACoA were very painful for me. When other members expressed anger, I wanted to run. Eventually, however, their stories of physical, sexual and verbal abuse put me in touch with my feelings of shame, fear and guilt. I discovered that because of what had happened to me as a child, I had been conditioned to become a fear-based personality called Tony A.

How It
All Began

CHAPTER 2

In New York City, in 1977, a small group of young people in their late teens began to grow dissatisfied with their experiences in Al-Anon and Alateen. These groups just weren't meeting their needs as children of alcoholics. Out of frustration they decided to form their own special-purpose self-help recovery group. This was the first step toward what would one day become a worldwide organization called Adult Children of Alcoholics or ACoA.

All these young people were products of alcoholic households. In sharing their stories with one another, they discovered that they found it very difficult to relate to, or identify with, the adult members of Al-Anon, most of whom were spouses of alcoholics. To these young people the older Al-Anon members represented one of their own family members with whom they struggled on a daily basis — the co-alcoholic (or co-dependent) parent who takes on many of the characteristics of the alcoholic in the family.

These young people recognized that they had many unhealthy survival techniques in common, and reasoned that their recovery needs could best be served by forming a special group that was not dominated by parental figures. They all agreed that such a distancing process would be essential to their recovery efforts.

7

For their first meeting they found a small conference room at the Brinkley Smithers Foundation headquarters, adjacent to Roosevelt Hospital in New York City. Though the group was developing a different stance concerning the nature of their alcoholic family problem and the recovery approach, they felt that some form of linkage with a national self-help organization would be beneficial. So, to attract additional members, they registered with Al-Anon as the Hope for Adult Children of Alcoholics group.

Shortly after the group started, one of its members, Cindy, heard me share at an Al-Anon meeting. In my sharing I mentioned that I had grown up in a household with two alcoholic parents. Much of what I discussed focused on the destructive attitudes and behavior that I had learned in my alcoholic family. At the close of the meeting—and despite the fact that I was almost 30 years older than their oldest member—Cindy invited me to come and share with the new ACoA group.

A few days later I attended their meeting and shared my story. I talked primarily about what it had been like for me to grow up in an insane household where alcoholism was king. I told them about how I thought I had developed many of my inappropriate and harmful behavior patterns to protect myself as a child. In recent years I had pretty carefully explored some of the crazy behavior of my alcoholic family, and I was quite vocal in my belief that most of my present-day problems could be traced back to the family chaos of my childhood years. I was able to describe in detail some of the damaging personality traits that had run my life for so many years.

When the other members of this fledgling group began to share their painful experiences and family secrets, I felt very much at home. A whole new dimension of recovery was opening up to me, and I promptly joined the group.

When I think back to those early beginnings, it strikes me that I was in a very vulnerable position. While these young people readily warmed to my ACoA personality, a few of them, who had alcoholic fathers, were somewhat apprehensive about me because of my own difficulties with alcohol. Since my pain and anguish were as genuine as theirs, however, most chose to accept me. Nonetheless I did feel their uncertainty and reluctantly saw that for some I represented an authoritarian parent.

In The Beginning

In the early days of ACoA we were grappling with the following issues:

- We were not at all sure just what it was we wanted to accomplish or how to go about it.
- We were very small; the first group formed had only five or six members.
- Our primary aim was to gain some measure of relief from current emotional problems that we felt were largely attributable to being brought up in an alcoholic home.
- The members of the group found it very difficult to trust and relate to authority figures or those we perceived to be professionals or experts in the field of human behavior. At some deep level we knew we had to be responsible for our own growth and recovery.
- All of us strongly believed that we needed a special and protected forum where we could safely share and experience our often overwhelming feelings of rage, self-pity, fear and grief.
- The format of our meeting borrowed heavily from the recovery process and approach taken by other self-help programs, such as Alcoholics Anonymous and Al-Anon. Many early ACoA members had prior involvement with these programs.

The format in those early meetings was pretty experimental. Usually a member would be asked to share his or her alcoholic upbringing story with the group. There was so much hurt and pain in those early stories that everyone would get upset, cry or just feel terribly unsettled. We finally voted not to have the leader describe in detail the family saga but just to discuss what had happened during the past week, within the context of the problems that seemed most troubling.

No matter how we tried to limit or guide the group input, however, the anguish and rage inevitably emerged.

Without understanding the process very well, we had begun opening ourselves up. Unfortunately we did not know what to do with all these raw feelings, and at the conclusion of each meeting most of us had to make a special effort to shut down our feelings. During the meeting we had experienced a safe, understanding environment. For one or two hours we had been able to talk openly about some common issues, unload feelings of rage and betrayal and receive loving, accepting support from fellow members. It was hard to return to a normal level of interaction.

Group attendance suffered mightily from this excess of strong feelings. Many found the sharing too intense and intrusive and some of the group members felt too threatened to continue attending. We began to flounder in our attempt to seek direction and purpose.

Within a few months the group had dwindled to just three members, and we were so discouraged, we wanted to give up. But I asked that we give it one more chance. I suggested we continue for at least one more week, during which I would make an effort to enlist people whom I knew had been brought up in alcoholic homes. Reluctantly they agreed to hold on for one more meeting. I was definitely a man with a mission. I wasn't sure what I was trying to do. I guess my instincts told me that the ACoA meetings were helping me, though I would not have been able to describe just how at the time.

During the ensuing week I went to a number of AA meetings in various parts of the city. I talked about the formation of the ACoA group, and invited recovering alcoholics who had been raised in alcoholic homes to attend our next session. On the following Monday evening at 7 P.M. some 17 AA members showed up, along with the two original members of the group and myself. My last-gasp efforts had paid off: We had a functioning group.

Over the next month the group continued to expand and grow. Our new members networked and brought their other AA members to investigate this strange new group that focused primarily on feelings, and where people were encouraged to talk about the misery of their alcoholic household and how early behavior and survival patterns were blocking growth today.

The Problem/Solution

As spring arrived in 1978 a second ACoA group formed at St. Jean Baptiste Catholic church on Lexington Avenue in New York City. I organized it and also chaired the meeting. Attendance quickly grew to 35 or 40 members, who were mainly drawn from the ranks of AA, Al-Anon and Overeaters Anonymous (OA) recovery programs.

Despite all this growth we were still floundering. Our format and structure were pretty direct, but we suffered from a vague sense of purpose and a poorly articulated solution. Although we considered the 12 Steps of AA and Al-Anon to be our basic guide, we were still improvising. The content of our meetings was heavily focused on painful feelings, often explosive expressions of anger and recitations of the family soap opera that had disrupted our childhoods. We had no literature to guide or enlighten us except the general pamphlets and books of AA and Al-Anon. We had no written information that spoke directly to our specific problems. Moreover the therapeutic community had not yet identified and investigated the dimensions of what is now termed the ACoA syndrome.

Our uncertain direction and purpose led to our first crisis. One Wednesday evening in early spring some of the members cornered me and complained bitterly that the meetings did not have a sound rationale or direction. Their concerns were certainly valid. Instinctively I knew that specific direction and certainty are prized by people who have grown up in explosive and unpredictably abusive households. I also knew that, as a group, we did not wish to be merged with AA or Al-Anon. In fact our second group had elected not to affiliate with any organization. We were trying to get at something very different, and now I was being asked to articulate just what it was we were all about and how this program could work for us.

The Laundry List

Clearly it was time to put in writing the general dimensions of our problem and some possible solutions. Until this point we had kept our special program tentative and provisional. But now seemed to be an appropriate time to go on record with what I thought we were all about. That night I spent hours thinking about the nature of our ACoA issues and how we could best resolve them. I knew I was in over my head but I decided to try anyway.

The next morning when I arrived at my office, I promptly set about writing down what I perceived to be the major problems and behavior patterns we had in common. To my amazement I listed some 14 items. I felt that I was receiving inner guidance and direction as I wrote the words. It was a strange feeling.

After completing the list I turned my efforts to outlining a solution. For this key element I drew heavily upon some of the AA and Al-Anon slogans and general guiding principles. I suggested that frequent attendance at meetings, keeping the focus on ourselves, feeling our feelings (and expressing them) and working the AA steps were the major tools we could use to recover.

I didn't set down anything particularly radical or progressive. Most of what I wrote seemed pretty basic. It didn't sound too therapeutic and it wasn't evangelism. It turned out to be a simple definition of who we were and what we might consider doing about it so that "we could get on with our lives in a more balanced and wholesome way." I then took this Problem/Solution to our group secretary, Chris F. She made some valuable changes in the Solution, and typed it up.

I presented this document to the group at the very next meeting. As I finished reading the 14 elements that described our problem, one of the members, Barry, exclaimed, "Oh boy, that's my laundry list!" So the group members promptly dubbed it the Laundry List.

This Laundry List and the Solution, also called the Problem/Solution, became the first formal document to explain who we were and what we hoped to accomplish. I read them aloud at every subsequent meeting. They seemed to help newcomers identify with their ACoA issues and the group effort, and the Laundry List also provided us with topics for discussion. (The Original Laundry List is on page xviii.)

Our second group was visited by two members of the national staff of Al-Anon. They reluctantly informed us that we could not qualify or be recognized as an Al-Anon meeting if we read the Laundry List or other literature not approved by their general conference. Since our second group was operating autonomously and had no burning desire to maintain affiliation, we elected to remain independent and not affiliate.

Change And Growth

During the next 18 months we continued to grow. Despite much turnover in membership we established a third and fourth group. Sometime during this period we started what was to be a long-term dialogue with Al-Anon to consider some form of affiliation. A number of our members also attended regular Al-Anon meetings and expressed interest in some form of national representation. During this time our meetings were frequently being visited by therapists and other mental health professionals who showed considerable interest in our new recovery program. Because our meetings were generally open to the public, we were also visited by members of the press, clergy and other 12-Step programs.

At no time did we see ourselves as pioneers of a new movement. We viewed ourselves as members of a 12-Step self-help program that focused on the special interests and needs of people who had been brought up in a family made dysfunctional by alcohol. In 1978 and 1979 groups began to spring up in other areas of New York City and in New Jersey, Chicago and Florida. Out-of-town visitors would attend a few meetings, grab a handful of our Laundry Lists and head back to their distant hometown ready to replicate the simplified recovery format that we presented to members.

Soon the professional community began writing and publishing books and pamphlets about the ACoA syndrome. Our efforts seemed to dovetail in a timely manner with the expanding "family systems theory" movement. All this new information provided us with much-needed insights that shed important light on the special nature of our illness.

Awareness of the ACoA self-help groups took a quantum leap forward because of the selfless efforts of one of our regular St. Jean Baptiste members, Jack E., a 20-year veteran of another 12-Step program. Jack moved to Los Angeles and, in true missionary style, he started the first West Coast ACoA groups. In less than a year there were many more ACoA groups all over Southern California. And with this effort ACoA became a nationwide self-help program.

On a personal level the program had helped me immensely. But I began to fear that my leadership role was creating in me a somewhat overinflated ego. I asked my Higher Power for guidance about what I should do. Shortly thereafter I stepped aside as meeting chairperson and took a much more comfortable seat in the back row of the meeting rooms.

CHAPTER 3

What Is ACoA All About?

What Is ACoA?

Adult Children of Alcoholics is a worldwide self-help recovery fellowship that speaks directly to the problems experienced by men and women who were brought up in a family system crippled by alcoholism. Despite much publicity in the media and dozens of recent books, many people who grew up in an alcoholic household are unaware that alcoholism is an illness that affects all family members—no one escapes without some scars. For millions, then, becoming knowledgeable about the effects of the illness is an important first step. An individual must come to the realization that growing up in an alcoholic environment leads directly to taking on many of the characteristics of the illness.

Until recently most people were unaware that everyone in an alcoholic household suffers some kind of emotional damage. Children of alcoholic parents are forced into an abnormal existence characterized by physical, verbal and emotional abuse, concealment, repression, stuffed feelings, chronic anxiety and continued betrayal.

As these children mature — that is, manage to survive — they develop a whole series of defenses that temporarily shield them from the brawling or muted insanity of their home life.

15

Such defenses as hypervigilance, deep distrust, inability to express feelings, depression, fear of authority figures and a compelling need to control events and people are just a few of the lifestyle tactics that children of alcoholics carry with them into maturity. As adults they are confused and often deeply distressed when they see themselves continuing to act out in emotionally unhealthy ways that they learned from their parents.

Those of us who grew up in an alcoholic environment need to understand very clearly that our family was caught up in a conflict that took on many of the elements of open warfare. Whether the battles were loud and calamitous or silent and deadly, they all produced emotional stress in the smallest of victims — the children. The tragedy is that the stress and hurt and agony didn't get processed and discharged. Most of us tried to bury it deep, to ignore it, to pretend it didn't hurt or didn't matter. Over the years all the buried, concealed misery festered. Some of us tried to rebel early, some later; and many of us never had the opportunity to shed our lost, stuffed, frightened selves.

As children most of us felt trapped and helpless, unable to establish a separate self. We weren't valued by our parents, and as adults we find it increasingly difficult to accept and nurture ourselves. But even more troubling are the frustrations and difficulties we have in our relationships with others and in our careers. Rarely do we have satisfying, healthy relationships with those near to us, and most of our friendships suffer from distorted thinking, dependency or domination.

ACoAs seem to have considerable trouble establishing intimate, mutually nourishing relationships. This is not surprising, since we had no healthy intimacies to observe and learn from in our childhood. Physical beatings, scathing criticism, sexual abuse and raging tyranny certainly did not help us comprehend the qualities and characteristics that create healthy intimacy.

In ACoA we learn that real intimacy and caring friendships can never flourish in the soil of self-loathing. Early in life, however, we were taught that we were unacceptable. We were told over and over again how terribly flawed we were. Our parents and other family members virtually created our negative sense of self-worth. Our real task as adults is to change how we think of ourselves. We begin this process when we join the ACoA recovery program.

ACoA is available to all who are interested. The focus is on reconstruction, change, healing, nurturing — and a willingness to surrender old ineffective ways of dealing with life's problems. By learning about the dimensions of our illness and the ways in which it continues to have a powerful influence on our lives, we can begin the process of change. We gain insight into the ways in which we have contributed to the current unmanageability of our lives. We begin to see how powerless we have been over the destructive force of the illness.

The ACoA program is about people, human contact and sharing. Recovery involves attending meetings, listening, sharing, learning and taking action. Most of us have tried in vain to understand where we were going wrong by studying an endless library of self-help books and attending lectures by professionals. Despite our efforts these activities never seemed to produce lasting, positive results. Why? Perhaps it's because an individual who is trapped in denial or resistance has very little possibility of producing substantive change.

Most effective change requires intensive exposure to the problems involved and a consistent effort to apply sound, sensible actions to the issues. Change and recovery seldom yield to solitary, infrequent, isolated effort. Self-help recovery programs bring success because they ask that the individual join with others who have common suffering. These programs invite the individual to suspend judgment, become teachable, open up to others, re-experience the early pain, take specific positive actions and develop faith in the process and a spiritual path.

The program demands nothing: The process is always voluntary. It requires a willingness to consider change, and a commitment to take healthy actions. The deeper your involvement, the greater the recovery. Fence-sitters derive very little of sustaining value. The primary law that operates in the realm of self-recovery is that the more you work the program, the more it will work for you.

How Does ACoA Work?

ACoA is people helping people. It is a 12-Step self-help recovery program with a structure, a series of well-defined issues and some proven recovery principles and guidelines.

Much of the early effort involves attending meetings and becoming familiar with the nature of the illness; learning to share with others on a consistent basis; and discovering some of the early actions newcomers take to initiate recovery. The program can be seen as a series of recovery efforts:

- Early awareness of the nature of the illness.
- Identification with the destructive behavior patterns that ACoAs have in common.
- Developing a feeling of safety and security about the meetings and fellow members.
- Developing a willingness to sit with and re-experience painful feelings that come from childhood.
- Sharing with the group about family secrets, shame, harmful behavior patterns and new unsettling feelings about childhood trauma.
- Intensive study of some of the valuable information and self-help books that deal with the ACoA syndrome.
- Developing friends among group members, active group participation and selection of a sponsor.
- Study of the ACoA 12 Steps of recovery for guidance and direction.
- Development of some form of belief or faith in a spiritual path.
- Assessment (in writing) of the major issues and destructive behavior patterns that are causing difficulty.
- Discussing these issues and problems with a sponsor or ACoA friends and developing a practical, workable program of action to resolve them.
- Applying the ACoA 12 Steps of recovery and the ACoA Solution to personal problems.
- Sharing the results of these efforts with a sponsor, friends and a Higher Power.
- Becoming willing to be held accountable by a sponsor and friends for following through on all major changes in behavior and beliefs.
- Adapting the ACoA program to all aspects of life, particularly to relationships and work.
- Developing a belief in the value of following a spiritual path in human endeavors.

Please keep in mind that the process of recovery varies considerably from person to person. The elements listed above are only rough guideposts that illustrate a general sequence of recovery events.

Early recovery is usually quite difficult for most ACoAs — even for those with other 12-Step recovery program experiences. One reason is that there are many different recovery issues involved. No two members are necessarily battling the same ghosts, since each member was brought up in a uniquely troubled family system. We all have much in common, but the specific ways we act out can vary. For one member an overwhelming dependency and fear of abandonment may be the major issue. For another member a controlling, abusive, suspicious manner may lead to a particularly troubling series of problems that destroys intimacy.

Some common threads run throughout all these different ways of approaching, controlling or reacting to life. These are described in detail in the Problem/Solution. This brief information piece was designed to answer the frequent and insistent inquiries: "Well, just how does ACoA work?" "How am I supposed to get better?" "What do I have to do?" "What is really wrong with me?" "Can I really recover from all this craziness?"

Early on in ACoA we recognized the critical importance of a safe and supportive environment where we could all share openly. Many of us found that opening up and expressing our real, authentic feelings was a frightening prospect. Most of us had been heavily censored as children. Our feelings were attacked, discounted or ignored. Now we were encouraging each other to be authentic and to reveal what we had so long edited or suppressed. We knew that we had to create a new kind of open forum where each member could share the special pain and anguish that comes to us when we begin to re-experience the feelings of rage, grief, fear and abandonment that we stuffed during our dismal and distressing childhoods.

When I constructed what I felt were the basic elements of a solution to our many and varied problems, I was guided by four principles:

1. Like our parents, we too were powerless victims of the disease of alcoholism.
2. By joining with others in a safe and loving environment, we could explore the ways in which the illness still affects us and gain a new clarity concerning it.
3. In ACoA the focus is inward and involves re-experiencing painful childhood feelings. Most of us have to revisit emotionally the anguish and confusion that so affected

us. A series of recovery steps is available to assist ACoAs on this journey.

4. ACoA is a spiritually based recovery program. Members are invited to look to a power greater than themselves as a helping force for recovery.

Who We Are

If you are questioning the impact of the illness on your life, you may find the following section helpful. ACoAs are the innocent victims of an all-encompassing illness that strikes any family suffering from the effects of parental alcoholism. In an alcoholic household the emotional dynamics are generally destructive to all family members. Too often the atmosphere is one of violence, denial, fear, abandonment, brutal indifference, seething scorn, inconsistency and betrayal—or a combination of these elements.

Turbulence of this sort, if endured for many years, invariably leads to some form of psychic numbing. Spontaneity and vulnerability get pushed aside by rigid defenses. Our feelings and emotions get stuffed and often covered over by denial and a powerful need to control. As trapped victims we adjust as best we can to the insane, unpredictable behavior of the entire family. As young children ACoAs learn a set of injunctions that are destined to keep us trapped in the illness for many years. Claudia Black has termed these:

• Don't Talk
• Don't Trust
• Don't Feel

As emotionally abandoned children these three responses were at the core of our survival techniques—we used them over and over whenever the family drama became too intense and uncontrollable. Even more destructive was the way that this behavior shaped our beliefs about life and people around us. We saw nothing was safe, certain or secure. We were always at risk. By following these harsh rules and directives we came close to being "buried alive" by our illness. When we finally left our alcoholic family we seemed destined to feel the seemingly endless negative consequences of the sick lessons we were taught in an insane and unloving family environment.

As ACoAs we have many problems in common, but our problems can be dealt with. The most universal or frequently experienced of these problems are described in the ACoA Laundry List (page xviii).

The Nature Of Our Problems

The typical adult child of an alcoholic has a number of troubling and distressing issues. This is understandable given the toxic nature of our early family life. The unique combination of problems that ACoAs must deal with presents a special challenge to the self-help recovery process. While most programs concentrate on a single problem such as alcohol, food or gambling, the ACoA program addresses a broad spectrum of difficulties ranging from deep fear of intimacy, to people pleasing, to extreme guilt when standing up for one's beliefs.

In the ACoA program the focus is on understanding, accepting and eventually changing our self-defeating behavior. In our recovery most of us have to contend with many kinds of entrenched behavior:

- Stuffing our feelings and/or being unable to express them.
- Going to great lengths to avoid feelings of abandonment and rejection.
- Isolating and being fearful of people, especially authority figures.
- Acting as people-pleasers and losing our identity in the process.
- Experiencing guilt feelings whenever we stand up for ourselves.
- Reacting rather than acting.

Even more limiting is the fact that many ACoAs tend to live life from the viewpoint of victims and are drawn to people with similar lifestyles. In recovery ACoAs learn that in their childhood years they were indeed the most innocent of victims. They were deeply harmed, but the damage is not irreparable. ACoA meetings put us in touch with who we really are.

When a newcomer to ACoA reads the Laundry List and recognizes how accurately it describes his or her life, a new awareness is born. It's like spirit calling to spirit. The newcomer hears a message of hope. Some have said that the Laundry List is like a child calling out to a child for support. Most newcomers quickly identify with both the elements of the Laundry List and also with the sharing of the ACoA group. On a fundamental level they come to realize that part of the process of recovery involves finding themselves through the sharing of others, and eventually through their own participation. Newcomers listen and begin to understand that for the first time in their lives they have a real chance to recover and be whole. They have an opportunity to experience supportive, nonpunishing, nonjudgmental family activity.

Like everyone else in the world, ACoAs need to be free to reveal what is happening to them and where they are in their life journey — without having to edit or conceal. For years or decades many ACoAs have, out of a sense of self-preservation, carefully guarded their thoughts and feelings. ACoA helps to dissolve the resistance and dispel the loneliness and isolation that blocked us.

Over the years people in self-help programs have suggested that a workable solution can only come out of an accurate definition of the problems. The Laundry List seems to be a reasonably precise depiction of the nature of our problems, and members feel that it is beneficial to the group to have this list of problems read at the beginning of each meeting. It sharpens everyone's focus, creates an invisible but palpable bond and encourages the process of opening up to the painful feelings within.

Feelings

Most ACoAs are masters at avoidance of feelings. We will go to great lengths not to feel our feelings. It's really difficult for ACoAs to grasp the reality that feelings are neither good nor bad, but experiencing them fully is essential to the process of recovery. This is especially hard because most recovery programs operate on the premise that the individual attends meetings to feel better. But in ACoA, when we go to meetings, we are more likely to feel worse because we are being opened up to strong feelings.

The members of an alcoholic family learn to feel shame for what they are and guilt for what they do, and this is an ever-present theme in ACoA sharing. Like other ACoAs, I had to learn that what I feel about myself and how I perceive myself isn't necessarily accurate. In my early days I had a terrible time with my estimate of myself. My angry self-loathing was engaged in a fierce struggle with the recovery process. My parents' definition of me needed to be neutralized. I was desperate to discover the real me, but the harsh, negative attitudes I clung to about myself formed an almost impenetrable barrier. I felt that there was something so wrong with me that I needed to be obliterated. This was only natural—I had been told again and again that I was terribly flawed and stupid. During my early years I learned to be hypervigilant—always outside myself, carefully scanning the external world for signs of danger to my brittle sense of self.

Part of my problem, like so many other ACoAs, was my ability to stuff and ignore the really strong feelings. Whenever I sensed any kind of abandonment or rejection I would distract myself by calling someone or by racing out to give support to someone else. Whenever I felt swamped with feelings, I would grab for something external to draw away my attention—a friend, a movie, a date, a party, television, a football game. It took me quite a while to understand that this seemingly innocent behavior was really part of my problem. I did not want to sit quietly and experience the turbulent painful feelings. I was still trying to escape from or blunt my feelings. I resisted the process of healing because it was so foreign to everything I had been taught growing up.

The Process Of Recovery

Recovery is complex. I'm sure no one in ACoA wants it to be that way, it just is. As M. Scott Peck so abruptly began his book *The Road Less Traveled*, "Life is difficult!" And I'm sure that if he were asked to describe life for ACoAs, he might suggest that life is doubly difficult. Our challenges as ACoAs are many. Not the least of them is to recover the self we abandoned amidst the tumult of an alcoholic family. Believe me, it can be accomplished. I know many who have done it.

Recovery is a process. It is often painful, time-consuming, confusing and most of all frustrating. Recovery is essentially a means of self-discovery and self-acceptance, and its ultimate goal is self-love. To this end the primary focus of the ACoA program of recovery is inward.

The program asks the troubled ACoA to open up and experience those awful feelings of fear, abandonment, rejection, rage, self-pity, sorrow—perhaps even wallow in them and literally mourn the emptiness of a miserable childhood. Most ACoAs resist this approach at first. We spent so many years stuffing our feelings that it's unlikely we will suddenly welcome them with open arms.

In recovery I discovered that I had to clear some kind of path through my self-destructive behavior so that the spirituality of the program could reach me and lighten my burden. Somehow I had to be emptied of all the sickness I had created. I desperately needed some clarity, and I intuitively knew that I could find some of it in a spiritual approach. I have never, however, been one who believed that there is only one path to recovery. There are many, and the ACoA recovery program is just one of those paths.

Newcomers to ACoA generally begin the journey by identifying with the common problems and relating closely to the experiences and behavior shared by group members. They see that we all have much in common, and begin to want to know more. One of the greatest tools available to both newcomers and regular members is the wealth of literature now available about the ACoA syndrome. A number of practical and insightful books have been published over the past decade by such forward-thinking professionals as Janet Woititz, Claudia Black and Bob Earll, to name just a few. Most professionals endorse attendance at ACoA meetings.

Awareness of our illness and how it defeats us over and over again is critical to personal recovery. The basic tools are the Problem/Solution, published literature and the inspired sharing of fellow ACoAs. Some meetings may be quite upsetting to newcomers. Strong emotions are frequently expressed, often explosively. These can be experienced as threatening, and may stir up long-buried feelings. Newcomers may also be witness to an intimidating level of anger and pain.

Early recovery follows this general pattern:

- Emerging awareness of the many ways in which the illness affected us.
- The surfacing of long-buried feelings and recall of painful childhood memories.

- A recognition of a powerful anger or sorrow at being robbed of a healthy childhood.
- A willingness to experience in depth the rage and eventual grief that usually attends a fuller under-standing of how, as innocent children, we were ne-glected or violated.

Unbridled rage and grief are usually difficult to observe and even more difficult to experience. Yet they are essential experiential steps in the recovery process. In my own recovery, and in the experiences related to me by hundreds of other ACoAs, the inward trip to recovery generally involves experiencing our feelings. It is critical that we open ourselves up to such frightening and threatening feelings as rage, depression and abandonment. It is essential that we sit with and experience whatever elements of pain and hurt surface.

Many times I wished there were an easier way. But I don't believe that true recovery can occur without a profound and inspired understanding of who we are as individuals, and the knowledge that who we are is perfectly acceptable and worthy of love. Until I commenced recovery I had been my own merciless judge, jury and executioner. I had never had a loving and nourishing model to follow, and I learned not to trust my feelings. In ACoA I realized that I had to make a beginning at listening to my emerging intuitive feelings.

React Or Act

I had been so conditioned to the role of reactor that I really did not know how to act in my own best behalf. Before ACoA I had always fashioned my behavior to gain approval, validation, praise and acceptance. How I felt about myself and my needs was of little consequence. In short, I was a consummate people-pleaser. In recovery this posture had to be corrected. When I started acting to serve my own best interests, I felt terribly guilty. I was saying yes to a healthy me that was beginning to emerge and it was all very uncomfortable. I had been desperately dependent on others and I didn't like to disappoint them. But I kept at the process—timidly at first, but with more conviction and strength as time passed.

None of these actions would have been possible without the loving support of other ACoA members. They supplied me with an awareness of the deceptiveness of my illness and they gave me unconditional love and acceptance as I made my troubled, erratic journey into self-recovery. I truly believe that a spiritual force was working through all those who were supporting my painful recovery. They offered nourishment rather than criticism. Though I judged myself harshly, they accepted me and related to my humanity. Slowly I learned to change my old attitudes and destructive patterns. I struggled daily to keep the focus on myself and my issues, though the urge to give advice and "fix" someone else was almost always present.

My need to control people surfaced early as a major issue in my recovery, as it does for so many others in ACoA. I wanted to be the authority, and sometimes I resisted the sharing and suggestion from others. I was telling others and myself that a spiritual force was my ultimate authority, yet I was loathe to let go of my efforts to control the people and events in my life.

Finally, through prayer, meditation, working the steps of recovery and consistent attendance at meetings, I slowly began to experience some recovery. My thinking and my behavior began to shift. Fear and anxiety, the cornerstones of my disease, began to lessen. I began to relate to myself and others in a gentler and more vulnerable manner. I continued to share at meetings and became increasingly more willing to sit quietly with my turbulent and painful feelings. In this way I gained some valuable new insights. When I felt confident enough, I began to act on my new awareness.

Through it all I had setbacks — many of them. Sometimes I would slip back to old forceful, judgmental behavior and make a disruptive personal assault on whatever or whomever was confronting me. And I always felt terrible after each episode—something akin to an emotional hangover. I was fortunate, though, for I had a new family to turn to for help, not my intensely dysfunctional family of origin. Now I had the consistent acceptance, support and concern of my ACoA groups. They provided positive encouragement even when I was responding to some of them as if they were my original father, mother and stepmother.

I'm convinced that my recovery is coming about because of three key factors:

- My commitment to show up and do the work of recovery.

- The love, acceptance and encouragement of my fellow ACoA members.
- The grace of a spiritual power, who worked through other ACoAs to give me a new life.

CHAPTER 4

The Recovery Process

Family Drama

It's very important for ACoAs to understand that alcoholism is a family disease that distorts all human relationships — those outside as well as those inside the family. As the alcoholic parent or parents become enmeshed in the disease, efforts to maintain normalcy and healthy interactions between family members disappear. Love, trust and acceptance are the prime casualties of alcoholism. Fueled by neglect, abuse or denial, the family usually enters an unmanageable stage in which all members are in some way seriously affected. The desperate spouse and children all suffer grave emotional stress in their efforts to adjust to the impossible demands and destructive behavior of the alcoholic.

Often the alcoholic family appears to be functioning normally. This is because it is drawing upon an elaborate denial system to conceal the true force of the disease. Robbed of healthy, nurturing role models, the children in an alcoholic household adopt the sick behavior patterns that they witness daily. All too soon the innocent young boy who is beaten and viciously criticized by his raging, drunken father learns not to trust, to withdraw and to suppress feelings. He quickly recognizes that life is not safe and he begins to construct a series of inappropriate defense measures to ensure his survival. Ironically these defenses may include the same rage and criticism he got from his father.

Spontaneity, initiative and high self-esteem are rare qualities among children of alcoholics. Personality distortion can take many forms, and children of alcoholics are highly susceptible to those that involve rigidity, inflexible beliefs, isolation, flash rage and morbid guilt.

A typical example is the young daughter of an alcoholic mother who at an early age assumes the role of little mother and substitute wife. She buries her own healthy needs and exhibits an overdeveloped sense of responsibility—serving everyone else's needs except her own. She may compensate for her mother's outrageous neglect by feverishly cooking, cleaning, washing and shopping for the younger children in the family. She literally sacrifices her energy and personal development in response to the demands of the family disease.

Some ACoAs take years to discover that the family was caught in the grip of such a destructive disease while they were growing up. In many instances the family never acknowledges or confronts the disease. Instead they engage in a conspiracy to "act normal" while concealing or seemingly dismissing the insane drama motivated by alcoholism. Unfortunately, whether it is muted denial or open family warfare, there is bound to be some long-lasting emotional fallout that touches all members of the family.

How Parents Define The Child

Scientists and medical specialists state confidently that much of our sense of who we are and our perceptions of how safe a place the world is are established in our early formative years, before age four or five. We develop many of our most fundamental personality traits and behavior patterns during these critical early years.

Early in life we receive a constant flow of important communications from the people who control our survival: our parents. Through these daily broadcasts we begin to form some general impressions of who we are, how acceptable and enjoyable we are and how capable we are. At a deeper, more complex level, largely communicated through touch, we are told how lovable and valued we are as human beings.

In a healthy family environment the children are shown consistent love and nurturing; respect for the feelings and actions of all individuals is commonplace; the right to voice one's opinions and voice one's needs directly (without fear) is assured; and healthy conflict and confrontation are encouraged as part of the family communication system. As the child of two alcoholics I find this almost impossible to imagine. I am able to describe these essential elements in great detail, but I can't really feel how they so richly empower those who are raised that way.

Over the years I have heard hundreds of ACoA stories that described the sick and distorted means that the parents and other family relatives used to give definition to the vulnerable children of an alcoholic household. Physical abuse, beatings, incest, scathing criticism, public ridicule, abandonment, emotional remoteness, smothering control, scapegoating, silent scorn, tyrannical punishment and sexual intimidation are just a few of the pathetic crimes committed by the alcoholic family.

They really are crimes and—make no mistake—the children are truly victims. These early wounds cause incredible injury to a child's fragile sense of self-worth and self-esteem. There is no safe passage to adulthood where a family is struggling with alcoholism or other addictive/compulsive diseases.

One of the real tragedies of ACoAs is how we discount and rationalize this alcoholic behavior. I have heard some ACoAs dismiss the most horrendous neglect as reasonably minor. In our effort to survive we internalize much of the family brutality and give it a new identity—such as, "I only got hit when I really deserved it." "What's wrong with leaving me in a dark cellar for two days? It really wasn't that bad now that I think about it."

Our Common Behavior: Another Look At The Laundry List

When I wrote the original ACoA Problem/Solution, I prefaced the Problem section with a simple statement: "These are characteristics we seem to have in common due to being brought up in an alcoholic household." For months I had sat at meetings with other ACoAs, listening to them sharing. Out of those early meetings I managed to gain some perspective concerning the nature of our problems. I wasn't conducting a professional or scientific inquiry; I was merely participating and noticing how all of us were linked by many common experiences and a series of behavior patterns that was creating great turbulence in our emotional lives. I also saw that our current problems had their roots in the many ways we adapted and adjusted to the stress and pressures of our alcoholic family.

Although it is unlikely that one person possesses all of the common characteristics or behavior patterns, it's a rare ACoA who can't identify with eight or nine of the 14 original characteristics I set down. In the years since I first wrote them down, individual groups have made some editorial alterations to the original characteristics, and quite a few professionals and writers have excerpted, cited, embellished and paraphrased my original list to fit their particular needs. Here, however, are the original 14 behavior patterns — the Problem — that I set down in 1977. I've added a few present-day observations to them — hindsight brings such wonderful clarity!

1. We Became Isolated And Afraid Of People And Authority Figures.

For many ACoAs isolation and fear were the most natural, almost spontaneous response to living with angry, abusive, hypercritical parents. Our parents were our first authority figures, and they loomed large over us in an almost God-like manner.

Alcoholism distorts human relationships, and the effects of alcoholism are particularly devastating to young children who naturally seek love, acceptance, respect and consistency. To be verbally or physically abused during the most vulnerable and innocent years can create either a fear of, or hostility toward authority, and a hypersensitivity toward angry, oppressive individuals. Many ACoAs continue to retreat into isolation, avoidance and distrust of people and relationships in order to ensure survival. As adults many ACoAs found that their reactions to authority figures either put them at the feet or at the throat of those they viewed in this way. As one member said, "I either wanted to kiss them or kill them."

Acquiring a more balanced approach toward those seen as authority figures is sometimes a difficult task. Until we learn to separate out and see that we are reacting in the present in much the same way as we did in our abusive family, we are bound to have troubled relationships. Just watching one's typical reactions — be it withdrawal, fright or hostility — and modifying this response takes real effort; but it's an essential step toward recovery.

Don't expect that knowledge alone will miraculously produce a new set of healthy responses. For many it takes painful trial over many months or even years.

2. We Are Frightened By Angry People And Personal Criticism.

One of the most corrosive and damaging aspects of an alcoholic household is the use of rage and incessant criticism to control the family's behavior. For many ACoAs, abuse often accompanied anger. As a child, violent, angry movements and gestures absolutely terrified me. Our parents were unpredictable and out of control. We, the helpless victims, had few defenses. We were completely at their mercy and full of fear for our survival.

As very young children we were also painfully susceptible to the daily litany of verbal abuse. We were being "defined" by our parents and we had no choice but to believe what they were telling us about ourselves. This ugly pattern of verbal harassment caused many of us to feel great shame and an overwhelming sense of inadequacy. Spontaneity, trust and confidence fled before these repeated verbal assaults. As adults we may sometimes be revisited by these feelings of helplessness when criticized or become very distressed by angry outbursts. Continuous badgering of a child over many years can, unfortunately, lead to resistance in recovery. As adults our reactions to critical or even mild suggestions can be alienating or inappropriate.

3. We Became Approval-Seekers And Lost Our Identity In The Process.

Very early in my childhood I began to watch the expressions on my father's face very carefully . By doing so I could quickly determine what kind of mood he was in and adjust my behavior accordingly. My responses to my father were always efforts to keep him "happy." Whenever possible I used humor to keep him from escalating a sour mood.

Approval-seeking became a powerful defense mechanism that I used whenever I was faced with people who were potentially threatening or violent—and my father was at the head of that list. I believed at a deep level that if I could get people's approval, they wouldn't hurt me.

Today I know that when I fall into an approval-seeking stance — and sometimes I find it difficult not to — I lose my identity.

I abandon my natural self. The real me slides under the door because I'm concentrating on responses and behavior that will please another — not me. So I have said no to the authentic me and yes to someone else's wants.

4. We Either Become Alcoholics, Marry Them Or Both — Or Find Another Compulsive Personality, Such As A Workaholic, To Fulfill Our Sick Abandonment Needs.

If we make a careful survey of those close to us, family and non-family, it probably won't take too much effort to notice that sometimes we are drawn to, befriend or become attracted to alcoholics or other addictive people. Emotionally healthy individuals with a solid sense of self-esteem do not usually link up with alcoholic, compulsive or emotionally ill individuals. Sometimes the fixers and rescuers, who have very cleverly concealed their own personality problems, marry or couple with an alcoholic in a vain effort to gain control or self-esteem through the process of rescue.

Conversely many dependent and addictive people have been known to reach out for rescuing by turning to those who closely resemble their most abusive parent. While the rational world would expect a mistreated child to stay well clear of an abusive romantic partnership, experience says otherwise. Pain and abuse are familiar to most ACoAs and often they feel almost comfortable in an abusive environment or relationship that resembles what they experienced in childhood.

Alcoholics and workaholics are seldom capable of being supportive to another person because their compulsive/addictive behavior acts to block their feelings. For many the addiction is the way of not feeling the feelings. Thus a parent or partner who purposely gets drunk is making a statement: "I am now emotionally abandoning myself, my mate and/or my children." When we become involved with an addictive person, we are at some level seeking that familiar abandonment we experienced as children.

5. We Live Life From The Viewpoint Of Victims And Are Attracted By That Weakness In Our Love And Friendship Relationships.

All ACoAs are truly victims. We view and approach life from that posture. We are readily attuned to and empathetic with kindred sufferers. Indeed there is almost a sixth sense that guides our affiliation and socializing process.

It is quite natural for victims to be attracted to other victims. Identification is often almost instantaneous; and those of us who are fixers and rescuers leap at the opportunity to become involved in attempting to strengthen and nourish another unfortunate. We fail to understand that we often do so as a means of escaping our own pain and turmoil, in the belief that by putting the focus on another we will somehow solve the many ACoA issues that confront us.

Often we act out the role of victim over and over again. Being victimized has a bittersweet familiarity and provides a consistent identity. The challenge for ACoAs is to recognize the many ways in which we perpetuate the behavior of a victim, sell ourselves short or discount our personal value.

Once we are aware of our sabotage efforts we can slowly begin the task of making healthy decisions that move us steadily away from the distress of low self-esteem. It's not an easy task but it does become less difficult with daily practice. Victims usually feel helpless about their lives. Healthy, esteem-building actions bring a more positive outlook and usually a more sensible selection of partners and friends.

6. We Have An Overdeveloped Sense Of Responsibility And It Is Easier For Us To Be Concerned With Others Rather Than Ourselves. This Enables Us Not To Look Too Closely At Our Own Faults.

When I take responsibility for others, I take the focus off myself. When I feel a compelling sense of responsibility for another, I'm no longer concentrating on feeling my own feelings. This behavior enables me to feel needed, wanted, essential and important. I now have a special worth or value. And when I feel needed or wanted, I feel full. As someone once remarked at a meeting, "Somehow I managed to serve everyone well except myself."

Since many ACoAs are driven by external approval, taking responsibility for another is an attractive way to gain approval and respect. The problem with this is one of energy depletion. Each of us has just so much energy to tackle life's problems and resolve them. When we use much of our energy to assist others, we are consistently robbing ourselves of opportunities to further our own well-being and self-esteem. Most likely no one will be particularly attentive and praise each of our little but important personal victories; helping another, however, can generate lots of attention, praise and gratitude.

This is not to say we shouldn't be of assistance and support on occasion. But we should keep clearly in mind that growth and change can only come from working on our own issues. This needs to become a primary task. To continually rush off to help others is to rob ourselves of a measured and perhaps accelerated recovery.

7. We Have Guilt Feelings When We Stand Up For Ourselves Instead Of Giving In To Others.

When I say "yes" to another person and "no" to myself, I feel at ease. But when I say "no" to another and "yes" to me, I may become troubled by extreme feelings of guilt. This is not uncommon among ACoAs.

As a child I learned that my acceptance was conditional and based upon my willingness to do what my parents desired. To refuse them would bring harsh disapproval. My efforts to assert myself were always met with great resistance; and I learned that my personal agenda — my needs, my desires — did not matter. My parents did not respect my individuality, only my compliance.

Very early in my life I found that I could be overwhelmed by guilt when I tried to assert myself. To hold fast in my own best interests involved risking the anger, dissatisfaction and possible alienation of others. I was never taught that independence and sovereignty were healthy. In my alcoholic household the focus was always on the needs and desires of my alcoholic parents. In order to reduce the possibility of anger or some kind of confrontation, I chose to suppress my needs and always be available to them. Even now, after many years of ACoA, I must sometimes contend with old guilt feelings when I elect to do something I consider important to me rather than doing something my wife or children want. The more central the person is to my life, the more apt I am to have some feelings of guilt.

8. We Became Addicted To Excitement.

As a child growing up in an alcoholic household I often found myself in the middle of a turbulent family soap opera. It was a household filled with tension, hostility, rebellion, guilt and shame. In some strange way it was both exciting and fearful, primarily because my parents' actions were so unpredictable when they were drunk. As a result I have a tendency to link fear with excitement.

My usual reactions to the insanity in my household were vigilance followed by a rush of excitement and fear. The fear became part of my identity. I became addicted to the rush of adrenalin, the hypervigilance, the dread of a family scene going bad.

This combination of circumstances made me feel very alive and allowed me not to feel abandoned. I felt that I was in the middle of, or part of, something very tense and vital. Unfortunately as a child I didn't understand that I was really engulfed in an alcohol-induced emotional windstorm that was making me sick.

9. We Confuse Love And Pity And Tend To "Love" People We Can Pity And Rescue.

Over the years I've noticed that some ACoA members have a certain way of looking and carrying themselves that reminds me of my own "wounded and lost" look. For me it was a manifestation of my state of internal confusion. The sick, abandoned child in me was crying out through my countenance and my posture. As an adult I tend to be attracted to the same woundedness, the soul sadness, the deep confused sorrow in others that I felt about myself as a child. I wanted to recue these people.

As a child pity was the closest thing to affection that I was able to experience, so now I have to watch that I don't confuse the two. In ACoA I forced myself to confront and work through some overwhelming feelings of self-pity. Eventually I had to wallow in them and re-experience much of my childhood sorrow. I had to surrender to the realization that if I felt great pity or sorrow for a person it didn't mean that I had to rescue them. My love couldn't make them whole — that was their task.

My effort to rescue people was an attempt to make them feel whole and complete. If I succeeded in "making" them feel good about themselves, then I could feel good about what I had done.

10. We Have Stuffed Our Feelings From Our Traumatic Childhoods And Have Lost The Ability To Feel Or Express Our Feelings Because It Hurts So Much. (Denial)

Fairly early in my childhood my feelings became so raw, so painful, so intense that I began to discount them and stuff them. In ACoA I discovered that my deepest reactions to abuse and abandonment, rejection and scorching ridicule, were carefully stuffed away in my subconscious. As events in my home became more and more unbearable I just buried the feelings that went with the incidents. In doing so I managed to construct an almost impenetrable shell around my early torment. I was unable to let all that early pain surface and be processed. It took a number of years of ACoA recovery to break open that protective shell.

Most of my childhood feelings came to light through experiencing similar confrontations and incidents during my early recovery days. As unsettling and awful to feel as these events were, they were just what I needed to open myself up to long-hidden feelings.

Even more damaging was my inability to recognize and know just what it was that I was feeling at any given moment. Long ago I had ceased being a sensitive, aware and spontaneous human being. I was a sort of a mechanical individual with a very limited range of responses and reactions that might almost pass as feelings—not a very healthy portrait. From what I understand about human nature, a person who has lost the ability to identify and express his or her feelings is pretty much buried alive in rigid inflexible behavior and incapable of experiencing life in a full and meaningful way.

ACoA meetings provide a safe and understanding environment where members can explore, identify and express their innermost feelings without the judgment of others. Meetings also provide a sense of belonging in which the vulnerable ACoA is accepted unconditionally.

11. We Judge Ourselves Harshly And Have A Very Low Sense Of Self-Esteem.

Children who are subjected to constant criticism and told repeatedly that they are "less than" are not able to develop healthy feelings about themselves. Our parents provide us with much of the framework and structure of our early identity. On a daily basis they define us as good, bad, lovable, worthless, helpless or inadequate. Out of this daily litany children develop a sense of who they are and the stuff they are made of.

In an alcoholic household the daily input is generally harsh, punishing and critical. Alcoholic parents verbally abuse their children in a variety of ways; but the result is almost always a child with a painfully low sense of self-esteem. Even the over-achieving hero children of an alcoholic household harbor troublesome feelings of not being good enough. Indeed their compliant achievements and heroic efforts are usually an attempt to compensate for the harsh inner voice that constantly challenges their adequacy and capability.

12. We Are Dependent Personalities Who Are Terrified Of Abandonment And Will Do Anything To Hold Onto A Relationship In Order Not To Experience The Painful Abandonment Feelings We Received From Living With Sick People Who Were Never There Emotionally For Us.

Parents who drink until they are intoxicated are emotionally abandoning not only themselves but also those close to them. Drunken parents are not rationally present for their own lives and cannot be emotionally present for their children.

Many ACoAs have shared that they would go to great lengths to avoid the terrible feelings of emptiness, loss and rejection that they experienced as children. This gnawing dread and uncertainty usually got converted into self-doubt: "What's wrong with me?" They felt that there must have been something tragically wrong with them that caused their parents to abandon them.

I think that a child sees abandonment in many forms. I was two years old when my mother died. I clearly felt that as abandonment. Every time my father got into a drunken rage and berated me I sensed that he was abandoning me. All were "little murders" of my spirit.

For many years I had trouble being alone. If I was by myself with no excitement around me and no people close by, I felt empty, abandoned and worthless. I needed constant attention and praise. I could not validate myself. I lived for the acceptance and attention of others because I felt that only they could reward me and fill the hollow, empty yearning. I did everything imaginable to shut out the feelings of emptiness. I constantly used people, places and things to distract me. My public behavior was mostly a desperate effort to conceal my inner poverty.

I was terrified of being rejected in romance. At the slightest hint of rejection, I would run. I was blind to my dependency. I desperately tried to control people and situations so that I wouldn't feel abandoned. Even now, when someone close leaves me for a perfectly innocent reason that has nothing to do with me, I still feel tremors of the old terror.

Of all the issues that ACoAs must contend with in their recovery, the terror of abandonment and the awful feelings of emptiness are the greatest challenges. For some it's almost pure torture to have to endure, alone, the painful feelings of rejection, loss or isolation. Unfortunately there is no simple remedy. Sometimes we have to accept the solitude, the apparent void, and slowly come to understand that we are not empty or unlovable. We will survive and we can have a happy and joyous life without being overly dependent or clinging.

13. Alcoholism Is A Family Disease. We Became Para-alcoholics And Took On The Characteristics Of That Disease Even Though We Did Not Pick Up The Drink.

When any member of a family is suffering with alcohol addiction, all who live in the household are affected and become ill. In some families the desperation and emotional turmoil is ever present, while in other homes the entire family may go to incredible lengths to put on a show of normalcy.

Regardless of the family posture, however, the disease of alcoholism affects everyone. The children suffer stress in countless ways. Eventually the overwhelming pressures in the alcoholic family lead to emotional disturbances, many of which have been described in this chapter. Appearances aside, all of the children in an alcoholic household become wounded and most of them carry those unhealed wounds into adulthood, where they tend to cause considerable distress in the work, home and social environment. No child escapes unscathed, though many are under the false impression that they have. It is most sad that so many ACoAs truly feel that they survived their childhood with only minor scratches and bruises.

Para-alcoholism is the transmission of emotional aspects of the disease from parents to children. Children who are exposed to the illness eventually take on many of the characteristics of the illness. It's a fact of life that many ACoAs resist before recovery.

14. Para-alcoholics Are Reactors Rather Than Actors.

On the stage of life the para-alcoholic waits for the signals and directions of others. The para-alcoholic is generally an other-directed individual who tries to determine an acceptable course of action based upon his or her perception of what will please and satisfy others.

The ACoA is often described as an adaptive individual with a very vague central self. All through childhood the ACoA was forced to adapt, adjust and respond to the needs and demands of drunken and often abusive parents. This child learns to react almost automatically, usually out of fear or need. And it is this response pattern, often driven by dependency and low self-esteem, that ACoAs carry into their adult world.

In the recovery process ACoAs need to learn to process uncomfortable feelings and demands without reacting automatically. What helped me with this issue was the technique of not responding immediately—no quick reply, no jumping into action. I forced myself to stop and think, which also gave me time to process the disturbing feelings that were bouncing around inside me. Instead of reacting I learned to temporize, to tell people that I wanted to think about it first.

Initially I was amazed at how people respected my request for time or my inaction. I learned that as an ACoA I had been programmed to respond in an unhealthy way to both sick and healthy situations. Now I usually take charge of my responses, and they are almost always guided by a healthy respect for what is appropriate and in "my" best interests. Most of the time I have stopped looking for validation and approval from others.

Waiting In The Wings

Adult children of alcoholics are definitely "at risk" as human beings. Recent governmental and private studies suggest that possibly 50 percent of all children raised in an alcoholic household become alcoholics and many marry alcoholics or other addictive personalities. The recent evidence also indicates that this generational pattern is also true for children of drug addicts and prescription drug abusers. In adult life many of us seem to be attracted to unstable partners and troubled relationships. The destructive forces lying in wait for the children of alcoholics are quite formidable, and adult children from these and other addictive environments need to be especially alert to these threats.

This leads me to some thoughts about the problem of alcohol and drug use by those attending ACoA meetings. I find it very difficult to believe that people who are using alcohol and drugs in any significant way can gain much value and nourishment from the ACoA program. Their escapist behavior is much more likely to move them into a nonfeeling, emotionally deadened space that is virtually unreachable. I would speculate that an active addict can gain little benefit from ACoA, and I also question the possible contribution of ACoA to those who are using drugs in a "recreational" manner. I don't think that active drug use and attendance at ACoA meetings is a successful formula.

Once, during a secretary's break at a meeting, I spotted two newcomers sitting in a remote corner quietly puffing away on their funny-smelling cigarettes. I thought, "What better way to avoid experiencing the painful feelings that may be waiting for expression. What better way not to be here."

While I certainly don't condemn the moderate and appropriate use of alcohol or the careful use of medication, I do think it is important for ACoAs—especially new members—to examine their current patterns of use of alcohol, prescription drugs, soft and hard drugs, and potentially destructive activity such as compulsive overeating, compulsive sex, gambling and debting. I'm convinced that most ACoAs are extraordinarily susceptible to all kinds of addictive behavior. All these destructive forces are literally waiting in the wings for most ACoAs.

As children and adolescents most ACoAs learned any number of ways to escape from painful feelings and the difficult challenges of life. Many reached for addictive substances or found relief in compulsive behavior. Much of what the ACoA was attracted to and used resembled the substances used by their parents. Thus the cycle of destructive behavior moved into the next generation.

My experience has shown me that people who have already fallen victim to alcoholism, substance abuse or compulsive behavior will make virtually no progress in the ACoA program as long as they continue their addictive behavior. They are simultaneously trying to drown and revive their lost child, and that is both futile and counterproductive.

A newcomer who is in a struggle with alcohol, drugs, excessive use of tranquilizers, compulsive food binging, gambling or debting is engaged in a wearying battle with powerful runaway symptoms. Until he or she leaves this battlefield and arrests the runaway symptoms, the ACoA program is virtually useless. We can't effectively serve two masters: We can't be fully committed to recovery and self-destruction at the same time. It's almost impossible to hear any loving messages when you are in full flight from feelings.

At a less obvious but potentially dangerous level, all ACoA members must become alert to the many partially concealed, seemingly innocent activities that may someday lead to an un-manageable life. I'm talking particularly about unacknowledged issues that have the potential to destroy ACoA progress and eventually cripple newly developed self-esteem. Often the be-havior is readily dismissed or discounted—a night of spirited drunken behavior that "came out of nowhere"; intermittent food binging while isolating over a long weekend; a runaway sex drive that leads to high-risk encounters, perhaps aided by a few marijuana cigarettes.

Isolated events such as these may appear to have little or no impact on an individual's well-being. Some people view them as harmless diversions and distractions that take a little pressure off a stressful situation or just plain "feel good." But these actions also enable a person to avoid feelings, and actions such as these have a way of becoming more appealing and more frequently visited.

Addictive/compulsive behavior normally escalates over time, but daily, life does not improve along with it. ACoAs are very susceptible to this behavior, and I have heard hundreds of ACoAs grudgingly admit that their behavior patterns include a number of budding addictive/compulsive activities from ciga-rette smoking to overwork to overeating to drug use. In time these presently harmless, "only once in a while" issues can turn on them and make their daily lives unmanageable.

The message is that denial can operate at many different levels and at many different points in recovery. ACoAs learned all about denial and concealment in childhood. Now we need to be sensitive to the possibility that we are attempting to belittle, discount or just plain ignore some potentially destructive addic-tive/compulsive behavior.

I make this plea for vigilance because even limited use of alcohol or minor compulsive behavior can so easily trigger pain-ful bouts of self-loathing, self-recrimination, depression and isolation. What may appear to be harmless behavior can readily undermine a person's early efforts at recovery in ACoA. Denial is a strong counter-force in early recovery; and newcomers to ACoA are not very familiar with the ways in which they are able to sabotage their growth efforts. For some the early path to recovery may require one step forward and two steps back.

Getting Started With Recovery

There are many roads to recovery for people who grew up in an alcoholic household. The ACoA program of recovery is one of those paths, but it is by no means the only way that an ACoA can deal with the emotional disturbances that have their roots in a dysfunctional family system. I am convinced, however, that the ACoA program can be of great benefit to those still suffering the effects of a turbulent childhood.

My own recovery began when I first sat and shared with a small group of people who were also raised in an alcoholic environment. I felt almost instant empathy. I readily understood the nature of their pain because I had suffered in much the same way. The circumstances and nature of the experiences may have been quite different, but my feelings and reactions to all that sick alcoholic behavior were very similar to theirs. This sharing and identifying was the beginning of my recovery process, and I think it is incredibly helpful for most of those who embrace the ACoA program.

My own personal recovery took a leap forward once the Laundry List was developed. Here were my major issues, listed on a single piece of paper, being read aloud at every meeting. Here too were some suggestions—the Solution—that I felt would move us all toward recovery. The Laundry List became my focal point. It showed me some real barriers to personal freedom that I needed to examine over and over again, and begin to resolve by consciously changing my attitudes and my actions.

What gave me great hope for the ACoA program was the realization that those issues that most troubled me were generally the ones considered most troublesome by the others in the groups. The Laundry List provides a reasonably definitive map of the troubled inner war zone, and the meetings provide a safe forum where people can commence the task of learning to trust, feel and share.

A Guide For Newcomers To ACoA

Newcomers to ACoA are often unsure about what happens and how to proceed. Here's the approach that I recommend to any newcomer.

Attend A Meeting

Attend a meeting and observe what takes place. Listen carefully to the sharing. You will probably identify with the participants' feelings and possibly the circumstances of their problems.

The format of most meetings centers around three key features:

1. Someone reads the Laundry List and suggested Solution at the opening of the meeting.
2. One of the members shares his or her childhood experiences and describes how those experiences have caused emotional difficulties in his or her adult life. Often the speaker then shares what actions were taken to change and grow.
3. The members of the group engage in a voluntary open sharing session. Members may discuss whatever issues they find most troubling in their lives and how they are dealing with them. At some meetings a single pre-determined ACoA issue becomes the focus of the open sharing.

I think it is important for newcomers to attend at least four or five meetings before they decide how helpful ACoA can be for them. If you live in a metropolitan area where there are numerous ACoA meetings (you can usually obtain a local meeting list at most group meetings), try to attend different ones.

You may find you are more comfortable at certain meetings than at others.

Sharing

At an ACoA meeting no one is ever required to share. Some newcomers have great difficulty expressing themselves, and ACoA members understand and respect this. At some meetings the sharing is done in turn, and it is quite common for some members to "pass" when it is their turn to share. Sharing is always optional.

Literature

Almost all ACoA groups make literature available to members. In addition to copies of the Problem/Solution, ACoA 12 Steps and list of local meetings, most groups display some of the more popular brochures, pamphlets, booklets and books that have been recently published about ACoA. When the ACoA program began, there was no available literature that dealt with the ACoA syndrome. Today there are numerous publications available at major bookstores everywhere. The newcomer is urged to take copies of all free literature and also purchase or borrow some of the more popular books.

A newcomer who is uncertain about which books to read should ask for guidance from some of the ACoA members. Most members discover that learning about the disease of alcoholism and how it affected them is an essential early task. It is vital that newcomers understand the nature of the disease and how it may be affecting them. Awareness is absolutely critical to successful recovery.

Commitment

Some ACoAs have great difficulty with the concept of commitment. This is not their fault. At some point they were taught that there was little benefit to being committed. In ACoA we invite newcomers to reconsider how they feel about making a commitment. In this instance the commitment we ask them to make is to their own recovery and well-being.

Although nothing could be more important than this, many people find the idea of commitment to recovery and emotional well-being to be either too threatening or too vague. Some

ACoAs can readily commit to grueling hours of training to run a marathon or throw themselves unselfishly into their business, yet they cannot give themselves permission to faithfully attend four or five meetings to explore the possible contribution of ACoA to their lives.

It is vitally important that ACoA newcomers consider participation in ACoA to be a central priority. Without a deep resolve, a newcomer is merely a spectator. Many members have said that when they first arrived at the doors of ACoA, their approach was passive. Fortunately they quickly came to understand that the ACoA recovery program held great promise for them, and they made the resolve to attend meetings on a regular basis regardless of the circumstances and other demands on their time. They became committed to change and growth— and they stuck to that commitment.

Regular attendance at meetings for a period of at least six months to a year is essential to recovery. Many members in large cities attend two and three meetings a week during their early recovery. The damaging effects of growing up in an alcoholic household just cannot be shed or dissolved in a few short months. It takes consistent focus, involvement, persistence and patience.

I sometimes think that ACoAs are especially attracted to the idea of the quick fix. They confuse awareness and knowledge with change. To know and understand about a behavior pattern is not the same as confronting the pattern over and over, experiencing all the raw feelings that surround the issue and actively changing one's actions and beliefs. I have spoken and shared with thousands of ACoA members, and one thing has become clear to me: Successful recovery requires solid commitment and a willingness to show up no matter what. We need to give recovery top priority.

Dropping Our Roles

Sharon Wegscheider-Cruse, who writes about adult children of alcoholics, has a theory that children in alcoholic households are assigned one of four primary roles by their parents: the hero, the lost child, the scapegoat and the mascot. The behavior attendant to these early roles is carried into adulthood and largely governs many of the daily responses of ACoAs. These roles are also evident in the way new ACoA members conduct themselves at meetings.

The hero almost invariably pushes to become one of the leaders of the ACoA group. Not surprisingly the heroes seem to be the driving force of the ACoA recovery program.

This type of individual is apt to jump in with both feet and embrace the program without too much resistance to personal recovery. Often, however, the hero's energies get diverted to running the meeting, rescuing and fixing. This was certainly the case for me. It took me some time to begin to understand my own control issues. At some point, no matter how valuable his or her input, the active hero must learn about the recuperative value of sitting quietly in the back row, relinquishing control and wisely replacing it with self-examination.

The lost child tends to blend in with the woodwork at meetings and needs to be encouraged to participate and share. Rather than fix and rescue, this individual is more likely to seek attention and rescue by others.

The scapegoat's impact on the group is usually obvious. Scapegoats tend to be rebellious and hostile. They challenge most authority figures and sometimes act out inappropriately. Their negative behavior seems to surface rather quickly, creating friction, fear and concern. Disruption of a meeting's supportive mood is always unsettling. While the expression of strong feelings is acceptable, over-reacting or personal attacks on others is always to be discouraged.

The mascot acts like the group's amusing pet. Mascots need to stop being distracting and people-pleasing, and realize they are suppressing fear and hurt.

Most people will find that they identify with more than one of these roles. That's normal, because we are complex human beings who sometimes change to fit our circumstances. However, you will probably identify with one role more than the others, and this is the role to begin to work on first.

Successful Involvement

What follows are some factors that I believe lead to successful involvement in the ACoA program. I know many members who have successfully used these approaches.

Learning To Trust, Feel And Share

Newcomers are seldom prepared to trust the group members or the group process. At early ACoA meetings it's more likely that they are following the parental commands: "Don't trust anyone outside this house. Don't tell anyone, ever, what goes on in this house; Your feelings don't count. Keep your mouth shut about what what you've just seen." Concealment, shame, avoidance, denial and silence are more apt to be some of the newcomers' approaches to their family secrets.

It takes time for many newcomers to see clearly that they are unconditionally accepted, that their secrets and shame are safe and that their sharing is respected and not judged. Group members encourage newcomers to share the long-stuffed hurt; to tell others about the misery that they witnessed in their childhood household; and to let others know how their early survival efforts have stayed with them in adult life.

Shedding light on all these hidden and shadowy corners is one way that ACoA members can begin to understand and accept the sickness of their childhoods. Little can be accomplished in the way of recovery until ACoAs come to see the nature of the disease and just how destructive it has been.

Many ACoA members must also come to terms with the actuality that they are holding onto a great deal of anger at both parents. These intense feelings of anger need to surface and be acknowledged. Newcomers will be best served if they can sit with and re-experience as many of those unsettling early feelings as possible. It's not a pleasant task but it is an important part of the recovery process.

Most children who grew up in an alcoholic home wanted to be loved and valued in a simple, healthy, satisfying way. The ACoA program provides an opportunity to test a newly emerging willingness to trust, be open and be vulnerable.

Changing Our Attitudes Toward Authority Figures

Our sick parents were our first authority figures. Often they were punishing, indifferent, neglectful, deceitful or inconsistent. Years of this behavior led many of us to be angry and distrustful in our attitudes toward and dealings with subsequent authority figures. Those who had early authority over us created a highly charged and untrustworthy environment.

We who were verbally and physically abused into fearful compliance must contend with the inappropriate re-enactment of that childhood anxiety or paralysis in our present-day dealings with those we have invested with the mantle of authority.

Whether it's a long-standing attitude of hostility and suspicion or one of fear and compliance, most ACoAs need to understand that it is quite likely that they will experience these feelings at the ACoA group meetings. It's also quite probable that they will have strong initial reactions to people they see as being in authority. It may take a while to understand that group leaders are merely serving the group efforts to the best of their ability.

It is important to recognize that inappropriate reactions to authority figures are rooted in the distant past. Most day-to-day conflicts are generally just modified re-enactments of old clashes and incidents.

Accepting The Group As Your New Family

Early in my recovery I made a conscious effort to be one of the group, a member of a family unit instead of a hero or group leader. I knew it was essential that I share and reveal who I was.

I began to notice that, in temperament and actions, some members resembled my father, my stepmother, my sister and even my wife and children. I had to monitor my reactions to these group members, constantly telling myself that they were not members of my family of origin and that it was inappropriate for me to judge, attack or be threatened by them. I pushed myself to act and share in as healthy a manner as I could.

As I learned to accept them and trust them, I also got in touch with all kinds of special new feelings. I began to feel really safe, appropriate and truly part of an accepting, loving group. All of us in the ACoA groups were taking what positive steps we were capable of in an effort to create and perpetuate an environment where we could all grow and change. I came to understand that I was a unique and cherished individual. For the first time in my life I began to value myself and see all the potential for an exciting, healthy, balanced life. I saw that fear consistently impoverished me, and I came to believe that love and acceptance can only flow through me when I'm not fearful.

Many of my discoveries came as a result of the concern and loving support of the group. As difficult as the concept may sound, it is vitally important for ACoAs to begin to accept the group as their new family.

Making Friends

Reaching out with a willingness to share is seldom easy, and it is probably most difficult for those new to ACoA. To ap-

proach a person, engage in an opening conversation, risk rejection, explore common ground and accept differences can be
very threatening and unnerving. It takes courage and persistence to start new friendships. It also takes some understanding of the ways in which ACoAs often try to control and direct
a budding friendship.

I urge every newcomer to try to develop friendships within
the group. Take time to discover those with whom you might
feel a kinship. Move toward those who have a way of behaving
or sharing that you admire. The more time you spend sharing
with people, the better the opportunity to understand them
and to develop some meaningful relationships. Take some risks.
Try not to be a loner.

Here a word of caution is needed. The overwhelming weight
of experience indicates that initial friendship efforts are best
directed, at least for heterosexuals, at members of the same
sex. Some developing friendships are started with the idea of a
potential romance in mind. While ACoA meetings have been,
on occasion, a mating ground, I think that newcomers should
focus on their major issues and not complicate their early recovery with ill-timed romantic ventures.

Granted, the urge to share can lead to a powerful closeness
and empathy, which in turn can create a strong romantic attrac-
tion. My observations over the years lead me to a rather fundamental conclusion: Try to keep it simple and concentrate on
personal change and growth. Romance and adventure probably
won't become extinct while you are working on yourself.

Willingness, honesty and openness can make the development
of friendships easier. Just being willing to put out your hand
and meet someone you don't know, giving a nod of recognition
or making a signal of any kind that you are willing to be friendly—any such actions can help the newcomer feel like part of the
group and someone the group members might wish to know
better. Being open and honest about what is happening and
how you feel are very special ways of developing trust and
eventually friendship.

Developing a friendship requires some vulnerability. My own
early experiences have shown me that becoming friends with
other group members is a vital recovery tool. They become the
core of an invaluable support system. Newcomers who hang
back, leave the meeting early and resist giving themselves a

chance to develop friendships are depriving themselves of an invaluable recovery element.

If I could make just one plea to the hesitant newcomer I would say, "Let go, and let others in." If you don't know how to let go, say so. It also helps to get telephone numbers and use them, even if it's only for a short, hesitant, "Hi, how are you?"

From group effort ACoAs learn new actions and new ways to respond to an adopted extended family. Those newcomers who maintain a distance or stay remote from the interaction of the group are avoiding a major opportunity to grow. Growth and change seldom come in isolation. They come through inter-action. Difficult as it probably is for many newcomers, I urge them to get involved, to make friends, to share their feelings with the group, to be available for after-meeting discussions and to arrive early and chat with the members as they arrive. Such behavior can be the beginning of the end of isolation.

Dealing With Judgments And Resentments

I know of no more corrosive and destructive mind set than that of judging people harshly or giving open reign to resent-ments. Critical judgments remove the vitality and spontaneity from any encounter and seriously limit a person's opportunities to experience and accept another. Most critical judgment blinds people to the good qualities of the person being judged and becomes a barrier to any possible friendships.

Similarly, the unbridled display of a resentment does not ad-vance anyone's recovery. Most ACoAs learned long ago that resentments were commonplace. Learning how to deal with them takes real effort. A productive way to handle resentments is to sit quietly and reason with the other person and express the feelings that are behind the resentment.

Try to avoid expressing blame and accusation. A resentment is generally a personal hurt that needs to be resolved *with* the person who triggered it. Blaming will only create new resentments.

Judgments are probably more difficult to bring under control because we are all guilty of critical appraisals of those around us. Sadly most of our harsher judgments were taught to us by our parents—we don't even own them. They were created by others; we merely respond automatically to certain individuals and behavior. Being willing to view people with an open mind

— to suspend judgment and just be with them in a noncritical manner—can create both personal and group harmony.

One byproduct of critical judgment is the destructive force of gossip. Restraint of tongue and the willingness to live and let live make it possible for groups to function effectively. Gossip is a particularly vicious way to undermine the spirit of acceptance and love. While no one is ever entirely free of judgments and resentments, we ought not be consumed by them. We can always strive for progress in these areas.

The Group As Your Family

I've always liked attending meetings, and over time the groups became my family. I was committed to them. Just how I began to see them as my family I'm not sure, but there it was. I could look around and see members who strongly reminded me of members of my family of origin. Sometimes during the sharing I could re-experience many of my early feelings of anger and depression, intolerance and fear. I could see what was happening. I was beginning to open up. Often only negative feelings came tumbling out. But in ACoA I was in a safe place and I knew that, despite what I was feeling, I was actively engaged in a healing process.

I was talking and trusting and risking in a new family environment where there was no judgment and criticism. We all shared our pain, risked confrontation and tested our new boundaries. With the Laundry List as our guide we all worked on our issues as best we could. Some of my early efforts were pretty limited. But I kept trying even when I was hit with miserable feelings of frustration, inadequacy and loneliness. I simply kept going, even when I felt I didn't belong and would always have trouble with the give and take of friendships. I was experimenting with new ways of responding, trying to develop healthier behavior.

Most important, I began to open up to the affection and concern of the members. They really cared. I lowered some of my defenses as best I could, considering my fears, and let their care and faith in me carry me through some pretty dark and uncertain days. The interplay at the meeting put me in touch with how fearful of people I had become and how I concealed it. But now I felt that I was being heard, and that what I said and felt were considered valuable. All the group members wanted to learn how to love and accept people in a healthy way and be appreciated and valued in return.

In my recovery I discovered that I was a lovable person who just wanted to be open and tolerant. I came to understand that, at a higher level, love can only flow through me when I am not fearful. In my relationships I had to see that fear and anger blocked my spontaneity as it did when I was a child. Now it was up to me to change my response in my new supportive environment.

During my first few years in ACoA I really had to struggle with spontaneity at meetings. My sensitivity, my need to control and my defenses were always working overtime to protect me and to keep me from being vulnerable and open to others. Once I had developed a give-and-take relationship with members of the group, however, I felt more protected and secure. On occasion this sense of safety would be threatened when someone I had grown close to would abruptly pull away and cease all contact with the group. This was very disturbing, because it could mean that the individual's pain was so intense that he felt he must literally abandon the healthy support and nurture that the group could offer. Even though I felt rejected and angry when this would occur, I vowed that I would never just "amputate" my group, regardless of the pain or frustration I felt. I became willing to stay put in my group, work it out and let the pain dissolve.

Working The ACoA 12 Steps Of Recovery

Many years ago a series of 12 recovery steps were created to assist members of Alcoholics Anonymous on their path to recovery. These steps have proven to be powerful action guides. As other self-help programs were established, they usually adapted these steps to their own needs. Al-Anon, Gamblers Anonymous, Overeaters Anonymous, Narcotics Anonymous and Debtors Anonymous all use the steps.

The 12-Step recovery groups represent a new way of living for many troubled individuals. The ACoA 12-Steps of recovery are uniquely for ACoAs. The AA steps are for the alcoholics—our parents. The ACoA 12 Steps are for us.

ACoAs should strive to make these steps an integral part of daily living. I'm absolutely convinced that I would have had a very limited and narrow recovery had I chosen not to learn how to love myself, take an inventory of my parents, keep the focus on myself and find a Higher Power to act as a loving parent.

For literally millions, 12-Step concepts have played a key role in the recovery from many addictive/compulsive illnesses and behaviors. They help clear away the damage of the past, and they are a resource that can lead to self-understanding, self-acceptance, self-love and serenity in a troubled and anxious world. Self-knowledge and change come slowly and often at great cost. Self-understanding can be greatly advanced by learning how our destructive behavior hurt us and the sources and causes of that behavior.

This is where the ACoA 12 Steps can make a positive contribution to sustained recovery. Following the steps can lead to a deep discovery of self and then to authentic loving. The following suggested steps of recovery give ACoAs a powerful guide to the recovery process.

Step 1. We Admitted That We Were Powerless Over The Effects Of Living With Alcoholism And That Our Lives Had Become Unmanageable.

When we lived with our sick family we had no way of avoiding the destructive forces of the illness. We were deeply affected by their insanity and sick behavior. Much of what we were taught as children now makes our lives unmanageable. We have taken on many of the destructive characteristics of the disease. We need to acknowledge that this is so, and be willing to commit ourselves to a recovery program.

Step 2. We Came To Believe That A Power Greater Than Ourselves Could Bring Us Clarity.

As children in a dysfunctional environment we had no balanced perspective or clear models to guide us. We had no opportunity to see a healthy, nurturing life process. With the help of our Higher Power, as we may envision It, we can begin to experience a healing and nurturing approach to life. Clarity, and with it a new richer understanding of ourselves, is available to us all.

Step 3. Made A Decision To Practice Self-Love And To Trust In Our Higher Power.

Instead of surrendering our lives to the sick parents that reside within us, we choose to put our faith in a spiritual power greater than ourselves, however we choose to define It. In my efforts to resolve the difficulties in my life, I recognized that I would have to accept myself and learn to nurture myself. I found that I could no longer give myself away to the needs or demands of others.

I used meditation and prayer to help me nurture and be patient and considerate with the vulnerable human being hiding within me. As a starting point I visualized myself as a very young boy and begain to nurture and care for that lost, frightened little boy who went into hiding to survive. One of my approaches was to sit quietly for a few minutes each day, repeating the phrase, "I love you, Little Tony." At first I felt foolish about what I was doing, but soon I began to feel a deeper appreciation for my inner child and what he had survived. Just as it is our Higher Power's responsibility to give us unconditional love, it is our responsibility to give our child-self unconditional love.

I also learned that this nurturing approach could help me heal the break with my parents. I could sit in silence and visualize my father as a frightened, confused, defensive little boy (and surely he was) and visualize myself hugging his little child. In my efforts to practice self-acceptance and self-appreciation, I began to discern healthy actions from unhealthy actions, toxic people from accepting and sensible people, positive situations from negative ones—and to take actions that moved me toward self-love.

Step 4. We Made A Searching And Blameless Inventory Of Our Parents Because, In Essence, We Had Become Them.

We examine, in a no-blame manner, the behavior of our parents. The ACoA's emotional responses to life are largely a composite of the behavior patterns of our parents. Growing up in an alcoholic household almost invariably means that we take on both the constructive and the destructive character traits of our parents. In order for us to forgive and accept ourselves, we need to see clearly who we have become and how much we still react to life as our parents did. No matter how far behind we may think we've left them, they've always been with us.

Many ACoAs have told me that early in life they vowed never to be like their parents, only to wake up many years later to see their behavior patterns and relationships were largely a carbon copy of their parents'. What confuses many ACoAs is the misguided belief that because the financial, educational, employment or social structure of their lives is different from that of their parents, then it logically follows that they could not turn out "like their parents."

As we work on this fourth-step inventory, two important discoveries may occur: One, we will come to see just how much we do resemble our parents emotionally, even though we may have steered clear of alcohol (and our family problems) when we grew up. And two, we may see few similarities in attitudes and behavior but come to understand the pain, fear, confusion and sadness of our parents' plight. In this comprehension may be the seeds of forgiveness and acceptance.

Step 5. We Admitted To Our Higher Power, To Ourselves And To Another Human Being The Exact Nature Of Our Childhood Abandonment.

Out of a searching and blameless inventory of our parents we come to see how we reacted, adapted, revolted and resisted— and ultimately abandoned ourselves. When we review the nature of our parents' illness, we come to see how many of their behavior patterns replaced our youthful innocence and spontaneity; we see all the desperate adaptations, all the frightened defenses we built, all of the repression, frustration and flight. Through these parent-taught mechanisms we truly abandoned ourselves.

All these harmful acquired behavior patterns we adopted are truly our childhood losses. We need to acknowledge them to our Higher Power, to ourselves and to another individual so that we can move toward a healthy self. The intent of this step is to help us recognize how we were emotionally abandoned as children and how we abandoned ourselves and became our parents.

Step 6. We Were Entirely Ready To Begin The Healing Process With The Aid Of Our Higher Power.

In this step we ready ourselves to turn to a power greater than ourselves. No matter how hesitant or uncertain we may be about the wisdom of such a move, we should keep in mind that healing can and does take place in this world and it is often propelled by acts of faith and belief. Here we are being asked to open ourselves to the healing help of a spiritual force.

Part of the process of healing comes from gaining an awareness of how much we suffer when we hold onto our damaging ways of living. We need to think in terms of preparing ourselves to shed the habits and traits that have so restricted our enjoyment of daily life. At this stage in our recovery we can make a resolve to open up and become more teachable; to embrace the opportunities and to move toward the development of a partnership with our Higher Power, as we understand it. No longer do we need to run our life by ourselves or in secret. This step does not direct us to take actions, it merely asks us to be receptive and willing to adopt a new approach to life.

Step 7. We Humbly Asked Our Higher Power To Help Us With Our Healing Process.

This is a powerful step. It requires both humility and participation.

Humility involves becoming aware that we really are not masters of the universe, and that in all probability there is a divine order that we can tap into. There are, however, three states of being that may get in our way.

First, we may believe that we were quite mature and sane, capable of adequately directing our own lives. Second, we may suffer from an overinflated ego that keeps us from seeing what exactly we are doing to perpetuate our problems. We are blind to any form of self-revelation or counsel by others. Third, we have no real knowledge or understanding of the specific steps and actions we would have to take in order to begin the healing process. We may be able to describe some of our problems and issues, but we don't know how to plug into the process of recovery. All of these can keep us from having humility.

This step also rests on a fundamental belief that we too can receive the gift of emotional well-being as so many others have through working the 12-Step recovery program. It is doubtful that all of these people could have recovered without some active request for assistance from a spiritual force of their understanding. Faith and willingness to seek out some kind of spiritual assistance has served many. Belief in a Higher Power is a form of humility. In seeking assistance, we move out of the driver's seat. This approach opens the way.

Prayer, meditation and a willingness to see and change our responses to people and situations are key recovery ingredients. Eventually we come to see that part of the healing process requires us to be absolutely ready to change our behavior patterns. We need not be alone in our effort—we can always call upon our Higher Power and the members of our group to provide support and guidance. The healing path can be made easier; but we need to understand that while we need not tread the path alone, we do need to make a strong personal effort.

Like farmers, we never will be in complete control of the growing process. We are asked only to do the planting and hoeing. The harvest will come from our Higher Power with the aid of our neighbors and friends.

Step 8. We Became Willing To Open Ourselves To Receive The Unconditional Love Of Our Higher Power.

In our alcoholic homes we were the victims and our parents were the aggressors. As we internalized our parents we became our own aggressors, unable to give ourselves anything but self-hate and self-criticism. Now we are willing to let go of the idea of ourselves as either victim or aggressor and open ourselves to the unconditional love of our Higher Power.

As we open up we are flooded with the warmth and love and acceptance we were denied as children. This infinite source of love is always available to us, waiting only for us to open the gates and let it in.

Step 9. We Became Willing To Accept Our Own Unconditional Love By Understanding That Our Higher Power Loves Us Unconditionally.

We became willing to give to ourself the unconditional love and acceptance we receive from our Higher Power. By actively working these steps we have begun the process of building self-appreciation and self-love, and affirming ourselves as full of worth and value. We are taking the important actions that will lead to well-being. We choose to put into play new behavior, new responses, new attitudes that will lead directly to a richer, more serene way of living. It is essential that we study these 12 paths to self-love.

As we learn to give love to ourselves, we also learn to give love to others, and to receive their love openly and easily.

Step 10. Continue To Take Personal Inventory And To Love And Approve Of Ourselves.

In this daily action step we monitor our actions and seek out those opportunities and situations where we can increase our self-esteem and self-love. We can use this step to correct our course in the event that we stray from healthy actions and begin re-enacting destructive patterns of behavior. If we see ourselves flirting with or contemplating harmful behavior, it's important to recognize that change must come from within.

We can ask our Higher Power for assistance and we can turn to our group for support as we struggle with those actions that bring with them self-loathing, resentments and guilt. We need to establish a new vigilance, one that centers on our behavior. This we can do by working this step on a daily basis: examining who we are and what we are doing this day to grow and change.

Step 11. We Sought Through Prayer And Meditation To Improve Our Conscious Contact With A Higher Power Of Our Understanding, Praying Only For Knowledge Of Its Will For Us And The Power To Carry It Out.

The primary goal of our spiritual efforts is to become open and receptive to our Higher Power. Our emotional well-being can be greatly enhanced through prayer and meditation. Becoming a channel for the will of a Higher Power can bring us to a new understanding of who we are and how we can lead a full and happy life.

Spirituality and faith are very personal matters. The ways in which individuals make contact with a Higher Power are limitless. There are many different prayers, many approaches to prayer and numerous forms of meditation.

Many people do not approach meditation and prayer eagerly. Some find it very difficult to sit quietly in a contemplative mood; they are much more comfortable with momentum and action. Others have long-standing resistance to the idea of prayer, which they confuse with supplication and pleading. A few people have difficulty with the idea of spiritual intelligence. People with these kinds of resistances are asked only to be willing to consider some actions that may bring them closer to a spiritual path or truth.

When I become open to my Higher Power, I strengthen my sense of well-being and feel in tune with my spiritual self. In such a posture I go beyond my self-centered demands and actually experience life on a more giving and sensitive plane.

A small note of caution: When I first began to actively pray, my conversation and appeals were focused on what I wanted and needed in my life. I was unable to get beyond the "I want" for some time. Slowly, however, I began to sit quietly and listen as well as pray. As I developed this "deep listening," which I consider to be the heart of true prayer and meditation, a new, richer peace and contentment entered me. I had begun to accept the simple concept, "Thy will, not mine, be done." And in so doing I freed myself from blinding self-concern and self-indulgence.

Step 12. We Have A Spiritual Awakening As A Result Of Taking These Steps, And We Continue To Love Ourselves And To Practice These Principles In All Our Affairs.

Self-love and self-acceptance inevitably lead us to feel connected with a larger universe. When we were victims in an alcoholic household we lost our authentic self to the demands of the disease. Throughout our adult lives, and especially in ACoA, we have been attempting to recover and cherish our authentic, spontaneous self. Through working these steps to the best of our ability and developing a relationship with our Higher Power, we can gain a wonderful new awareness and an opportunity to truly change. We can find a happiness and contentment beyond anything we could imagine. This does not mean that our life will always be trouble-free, only that we can readily and confidently deal with life's problems.

There is a solution beyond ourselves. By working the program daily and admitting we are powerless over the effects of living with alcoholism, we can learn to love ourselves. And when we do we are free to love others in a new, healthy way.

By sharing with each other we act as a mirror, reflecting our new growth and love. By using this program in all our affairs we can dispel the old destructive personality that so crippled our enjoyment of life. No longer do we imitate a normal life. Now we embrace it.

The Importance Of Accountability

Identifying Our Issues

A principal purpose of the Laundry List is to help define a way of living that can at best be described as troublesome, and at worst terribly punishing. For many new ACoA members, the Laundry List is an initial point of identification. Newcomers see in print some of their most unwholesome behavior patterns, their most painful responses to life, and realize they are not alone.

As they attend meetings and start to recount the distorted ways in which they adapted to their family illness, they begin to gain clarity concerning their early problems and the powerful forces involved. With time, many meetings and the working of the ACoA 12-Steps of recovery, newcomers begin to make connections between the desperate responses of their childhood and their current behavior patterns. Listening to other group members share current problems also aids them in gaining perspective about their own issues.

Your Own Laundry List

At some point during the early months of ACoA attendance newcomers should take pen in hand and make a list of the bothersome issues and behavior patterns that are most troubling to them in their day-to-day affairs — their own "laundry list." An excellent starting point is the ACoA Laundry List. For those who may be too confused to know where to begin and for those who might mistakenly see all current behavior as troublesome, the Laundry List is a practical and reasonable reference. The newcomer might consider circling those that apply and then listing them on a separate sheet in two distinct groups: (1) those that seem to be causing frequent or persistent difficulties in their personal and work relationships; and (2) those that are causing only occasional but significant disruption in their enjoyment of life.

In addition to the problems described in the Laundry List, members of ACoA may also identify other issues such as compulsive overeating, overspending, inappropriate drinking behavior, shoplifting, abrupt amputation of friendships, compulsive lying to friends and relatives, and high-risk sexual activity. They should add such difficulties to the list.

The purpose of this activity is to get clear about the nature and gravity of the troublesome behavior that may be seriously diminishing the joys of living. This is an effort to gain clarity. Such activity works well in conjunction with steps two, three, four and five of ACoA recovery. Step two, for example, involves the belief that we can gain clarity and understanding about our destructive patterns. Not all destructive behavior is overt. People-pleasers go to great lengths to satisfy others and maintain harmony. While this might be considered as an appropriate and friendly way of responding to the world, at a personal level, people-pleasing robs the ACoA of a centered and healthy self. In listing the issues and actions that cause us difficulty, we might use this distinction as a guide.

Over time the newcomer may add to the list as self-knowledge grows. Usually a searching and blameless inventory of parents' behavior patterns will turn up additional issues and traits that cause the ACoA complications. The effort at this stage is to build a portrait of unhealthy responses to what life presents us. The goal is understanding and clarity. Without a clear understanding of what is holding the ACoA back there can be no purposeful movement forward. Most people cannot really confront or begin to deal with what they can't recognize or understand.

At some quiet time at the end of each day, ACoA members should sit with their personal laundry list and try the following:

- Read each issue slowly and thoughtfully.
- Reflect on each item and determine whether the issue caused problems during the current day.
- Review the circumstances of any disruption or event that occurred, and review what or how the ACoA's attitudes and actions contributed to the problem.
- Consider what would have been a more wholesome response or action.

Awareness

The intent of the foregoing effort is to help the ACoA become thoroughly familiar with the nature of his or her issues and the extent to which they cause problems and upset. This review should not be seen as a time to engage in intensive self-criticism. A negative approach can only bring frustration and despair. The ACoA is being asked to review, in a noncritical and blameless way, how the troublesome issues got triggered, their responses and the results that occurred.

With effort the ACoA will begin to see that awareness alone is not recovery. True clarity involves awareness of the self-defeating patterns, some understanding of how the individual activates the problems and a recognition that certain efforts will be needed to bring about meaningful change. Fortunately no one is asked to do this alone. Other members of the group are available for support, and a Higher Power of our understanding is always accessible to us if we choose to seek spiritual guidance and nourishment.

Journals

Some ACoA members have found that keeping a journal is also very helpful. The journal might be divided into three sections.

1. A list of the most troublesome issues to be worked on.
2. A daily diary where the ACoA can record both successful and unsuccessful efforts to correct major personal issues.
3. A list of personal recovery goals that can be referred to on a daily basis. (Recovery goals are discussed in detail in the next section.)

I have found that keeping a journal or diary can be very helpful. In my own life I am easily distracted and tend to drift away from my recovery goals. Having these goals written down and reviewing them daily keeps my issues fresh and also keeps me focused on the positive aspects of my recovery.

Establishing Recovery Goals

This section deals with one approach to recovery that ACoAs often resist. Some ACoAs find that any discussion of recovery goals strikes them as too impersonal and mechanical. As living, breathing, vital human beings they feel the recovery process should not be reduced to some kind of exercise.

After considerable struggle I have come to believe that establishing some personal recovery goals, and putting them on paper along with some thoughts about how to achieve these goals, can accelerate recovery. I find that it's very easy to lose sight of where I'm going and how I plan to get there, and others have told me this is also true for them.

My first efforts at goal-setting were pretty limited. Fortunately I had enough sense not to bite off more than I could chew. I decided to tackle some of my smaller personal issues, because I knew that with effort they might clear up quickly. For instance, I "inherited" my parents' tendency to be rude and demanding of store personnel. So I set myself a goal of reversing this habit. When I went into stores I made a conscious effort to be pleasant and friendly. I succeeded on some occasions and failed on others. But as I made the effort, it got easier, and this soon ceased to be an issue with me. Starting with simple problems allowed me to see progress right away, which helped build my sense of self-esteem and confidence.

I found that it was important to draw myself a map of how I intended to tackle my issues. I really wasn't anxious to go into such detail. But I knew that if I didn't draw up some course of action I would leave too much to chance. If I wanted to be healthy I had to be willing to take appropriate steps. By then I was able to turn to my Higher Power for energy and resolve.

Someone once told the following story at a meeting, and it gave me a great image to remember: A traveler wanted to cross a dangerous river. The traveler was told he could row the boat and look to his Higher Power (whom he called God) to steer. He was also informed that, if he absolutely wanted to, he could take the helm and steer instead, but that God had a policy of not rowing! I always remember this when I am tempted to wait for miracles.

My recovery is teaching me one very invaluable lesson: I can not expect growth and recovery if I don't make a really sustained effort. Sometimes what I really want is a magical recovery, preferably one where my Higher Power wipes my slate clean in just a few months and I am promptly given the gift of emotional well-being. In this fantasy I see my role as being limited to some in-depth sharing. The rest would be miraculously done for me! Unfortunately it doesn't quite happen that way. I have to do the rowing.

I cannot overstate the value of listing your issues on a piece of paper along with the ways in which you plan to work on them. Recovery takes on more importance and meaning when you write down your goals and review them frequently. Troublesome issues don't get away from us so easily when we keep them in focus.

Other Common Difficulties

In addition to the problems described in the Laundry List, some additional ways of behaving often cause continuous irritation and disharmony. Chief among them are control issues, critical judgment, an overinflated sense of self, intolerance and giving advice.

Control Issues

The effort to control the actions of others, the environment and all manner of situations are often a problem for ACoAs. Taking charge, being in control, manipulating others, being bossy, bulldozing through—whatever the description, it is for many a constant source of concern.

Control issues generally involve the critical (and impossible) need to arrange life's events so that things are safe, secure and predictable. Often "rescuers" turn to heavy control. In rescuing they see that the rescued one is dependent; thus the rescuer has control and is not vulnerable. The rescuer can feel safe, secure and wanted.

Control issues began early for me. I learned as a young boy that by manipulating my parents with humor I could put them in a good mood and get them to respond favorably to me. It was my primitive effort to arrange things so that anger and abuse would not erupt. When my parents were angry, anything could happen and I was very fearful. So I relied on humor to protect me. I became hypervigilant, always watching for signals from the external world that could lead to criticism, hurt or embarrassment. As a child I became fear-based, and I found I could reduce this fear by controlling people, places and things as a people-pleaser.

Criticism

Critical and negative appraisal of others also can be very destructive. It serves no beneficial purpose and it can easily lead to isolation. Criticism not only pushes people away, it also draws attention away from personal issues.

A frequent quip in ACoA used to be, "I haven't got time to work on my own issues because I'm too busy taking everyone else's inventory." Growth and progress require both energy and concentration. Try not to waste time on the useless and counterproductive habit of finding fault with others—it can easily occupy all of your waking hours.

A leading marriage counselor cautions that the most destructive force in any relationship is continual criticism, and he instructs his clients that they absolutely must drop all criticism of one another from their daily communication. This is a powerful instruction that ACoAs might find helpful. Criticism can keep us all away from looking at our own shortcomings. For many it feeds the distorted need to be seen as superior to others. But what it really does is clearly separate us from others. How can I be open to another person and really hear who they are over the roar of my criticism of them? If one objective is to live in harmony with those around us—and work on our own issues— then criticism can only be viewed as counterproductive. As the preamble of one recovery program admonishes, "Let there be no criticism of one another."

Overinflated Sense Of Self

An overinflated sense of self can cause havoc with any and all kinds of relationships. Like most people I developed an image of who I was and how I wanted people to see me based upon how I was treated as a child and how I was defined by my parents. Consequently I acquired some pretty distorted views of myself.

Early in my teens I developed a kind of defensive arrogance, a posture of false superiority. These I used when I found myself in threatening social situations or in those instances where my demands for special attention weren't being met. I used intimidation to get me through many situations where I felt out of control and vulnerable. I flashed a certain kind of pride that kept me aloof from others. In ACoA these approaches often robbed me of a chance to be one with fellow members, for even in ACoA meetings it took me a while to get rid of much of the inflated self that had worked to keep me invulnerable.

Getting to see the nature of my unworkable self-images was very difficult. Like others, I had trouble acknowledging my defensive arrogance and pride. Before I was willing to give them up, I wanted something new that would keep me invulnerable and would continue to protect me from others and their reactions to me.

Intolerance

Intolerance — being closed to other ideas, approaches or suggestions — has slowed down more than a few recovery efforts. When a person's discomfort level is high, being open to new and different ways of living is often very difficult. Long-cultivated negative response patterns don't take kindly to the introduction of constructive suggestions. Many prefer to rely on time-tested reactions, such as pulling back, ignoring the issue and suppressing feelings.

Whatever the threat, we usually want to be well protected. Being open and tolerant of change involves letting go and surrendering. Awareness and knowledge of who we are cannot be forced on us, but ACoAs can advance recovery by cultivating an environment of open-minded willingness to try sensible suggestions and approaches. Flash rage and hostility can turn much of recovery (and life in general) into a shambles. Somewhere in our youth some of us may have used rage and anger as a defense or as a way of getting some of our needs met, but now it serves us poorly in most of the adult world.

Flash rage and hostility are not viable methods of interacting and responding. We need not stuff our anger; we can let it course through us. But we don't improve anything by exploding at our friends and family or fellow members. Some, I imagine, see anger as a power tool to frighten and intimidate. Explosive rage tends to be threatening to some ACoA members and is generally unsettling to everyone. Attacks of righteous indignation seldom further anyone's growth, nor do hostile putdowns concealed as helpful sharing.

I have learned that when I am filled with rage, I can employ a few strategies to help me cool down. If I am alone I write out my anger and rage in a journal. If I am with another person, I say, "I need to take some time out" and walk away. Another technique I use is to take slow, deep breaths and slowly count backwards until I feel calmer. Restraint of tongue needs to become a way of life for those afflicted with a compelling need to explode and attack in rage. Venting the rage and dissipating the hostility need to be done in a safe supportive environment— in a therapist's office, with a sponsor or close friend, or yelling at the ocean when no one is around.

Giving Advice

Giving advice can be a wonderful and mutually beneficial activity. Unfortunately in ACoA it can sometimes prove to be troublesome. We all know people who spend many of their waking hours dispensing advice, guidance and direction to others. Giving advice is often a means of avoiding the pain of one's own problems. If an ACoA adopts this advise-and-rescue role, you can be pretty sure that somewhere there is a good bit of deflecting or avoidance of personal problems.

One of the things I learned in Al-Anon is that the worst vice is ad-vice. Suggestions work much better. It's still a struggle for me to let go of this need. I'm learning to get my ego out of the way, face my own issues and work on them rather than on the sketchy and convoluted issues others may present to me. With the aid of my Higher Power I've learned some things about what troubles people and why, but I'm reasonably hesitant about advising others how to conduct their romantic, family or work affairs. However, since you are reading this book, you've seen that I don't hesitate to talk about recovery and some of the lessons I'm learning.

Enlisting The Support Of Others

Just about everyone in ACoA knows how difficult it is to reach out to others. A major fear is that those to whom you turn for assistance will reject your request, treat your request with indifference or (even worse) criticize your efforts. Fortunately I have rarely seen this happen. Most members are keenly aware that ACoA is a fellowship that involves sharing and caring. Love, nurture and support are freely given to the extent that the individual member is capable.

It's probably not too wise to approach a newcomer with complex problems or issues. If you happen to be working on the eleventh step of recovery, your sharing about prayer and meditation might produce only a limited response if you have turned to a newcomer for guidance.

Let's say you are having trouble at work. Perhaps your boss is on your case for tardiness. Rather than jeopardize your job or career, you could ask a group member who rises early to call you and support you in your commitment to be on time. Perhaps you are planning a holiday visit to your parents' home in a distant city. You haven't seem them in two years, you now have five months in ACoA and you are very concerned about how you will behave during the visit. By all means ask one or two group members if you can phone them for support during your visit, in the event that things get too strained or you lose perspective. Maybe you're feeling pretty secure but you just want some added insurance or a safety net. Nothing triggers reactive behavior and high-level stress like a visit with parents during the holidays!

I think that willingness is the key to getting the greatest amount of benefit from your group. Avail yourself of every positive attribute the group can offer. Not a few newcomers think that they must accomplish their growth alone. After all, that's how it was growing up in an alcoholic household: Don't trust others, do it yourself. Part of growth is in learning to trust others. And part of trusting others involves reaching out for support—especially when you feel you are on thin ice. I do it over and over again and it works for me. I had to rid myself of the awful tendency to go it alone. My fear of people, dread of criticism and feelings of inadequacy were always conspiring to keep me on a painful and potentially damaging solitary path. In ACoA we all have a chance to abandon the solitary journey.

Many ACoAs seek support from others in monitoring their stated goals. I know that left to my own devices I might never have completed the ACoA 12 Steps of recovery and I would not have taken such bold measures. Fortunately I had enough sense to understand that by myself I would accomplish little, but that I could accomplish miracles with the support of others and the divine grace of my Higher Power. And that's how I view myself now, as a miracle. But I had to reach out, to ask others to hold me accountable and responsible for whatever it was that I set out to do. I needed concerned and caring people who had a vital interest in my recovery and expected me to have an interest in them. In a larger sense, when one of us recovers, we all benefit.

In my early days I formulated my personal program for recovery. The ACoA 12 Steps and my own issues were sitting there waiting to be confronted. I allowed my Higher Power to steer, but I had to row. To keep me focused on my efforts I informed others about what I planned to do and asked them to be available for reporting and review. In doing this I ensured that I was no longer alone. I had made my recovery a collaborative effort. I could mess up on my goals, fall short, adjust my goals — do just about anything — yet they would continue to be there in a concerned, nonjudgmental, no-blame capacity. They listened, they made suggestions, they encouraged me — and above all they showed me that they truly wanted me to recover. So I grew and changed and am continuing the process of recovery.

Sponsorship

Many 12-Step programs endorse the concept of formally selecting a sponsor. A sponsor is an individual you can turn to regularly for guidance, direction and assistance in your recovery process. His or her principal role is to provide perspective, support and encouragement to the newcomer or sponsee. Typically, the sponsor has considerable time in the 12-Step program, demonstrates sound recovery behavior and is someone you respect.

The sponsorship concept works remarkably well, particularly in Alcoholics Anonymous, the largest and oldest 12-Step program. It has been a time-tested and proven aid to millions. One reason might be that a sponsor demonstrates concern, is willing to be supportive and above all holds the newcomer or sponsee accountable. A newcomer who is willing to surrender some personal sovereignty can benefit immeasurably. Sponsorship can start the process of trusting and sharing with another individual. Newcomers can profit from impartial, concerned and caring feedback.

Counterbalancing all these advantages of sponsorship are the few instances where the sponsor selected was sadly unqualified or perhaps too emotionally distressed to provide a sponsee with sound direction. In most instances I have heard about, the damage was not irreparable; a Higher Power seems to intervene and repair such ill-fated selections.

Sponsorship and selection of a sponsor are voluntary acts. No one is wedded to a sponsor or sponsee. Sponsors have a responsibility to be supportive, caring and enlightening. They have no mandate to be overbearing, hypercritical or abusive to those who seek their help. In those rare instances where unhealthy behavior occurs, the sponsee should dissolve the sponsorship. This approach also should be taken where there is too much friction or dissension.

Ideally sponsorship provides an opportunity for the newcomer to begin trusting and talking at a deep personal level. In sponsorship the newcomers need to be able to drop their defenses and begin to be teachable. For heterosexuals, the sponsor relationship is more effective if those involved are of the same sex. In any case sexuality should not be a part of the relationship.

The role of sponsorship in ACoA is somewhat clouded. Some groups endorse it, while others shy away from it. Since many ACoAs have great difficulty with authority figures, mentors or advisers due to years of parental abuse and inconsistency, I can readily understand the reluctance to embrace sponsorship.

On balance, however, I favor sponsorship. It has proven such a valuable aid to recovery in so many other programs that it deserves careful consideration in ACoA.

Seeking Professional Assistance

Some members of ACoA need more help then they can get in an ACoA recovery group. It's not unusual for some ACoAs to have a suitcase full of problems when they join ACoA. Some of the problems may yield to the application of the ACoA recovery principles, but others may prove infinitely more resistant to the ACoA healing process.

For these people ACoA group therapy or one-to-one therapy with a qualified ACoA -trained professional may be a wise solution. In the past few years, numerous treatment centers throughout the United States have developed intensive, on-site recovery programs that involve one- to four-week concentrated group and individual therapy specifically for ACoAs.

I don't believe that ACoA can or should stand alone as the only treatment for ACoAs. ACoAs need to understand that a full commitment to recovery will always benefit from consistent and frequent attendance at ACoA meetings. The development of numerous ACoA friendships, working the recovery steps and, where desired, some therapy, all can help.

Those who elect to undertake ACoA therapy will benefit most if they find a professional who is thoroughly trained in ACoA issues and the ACoA program. With denial and resistance so strong in our emotional make-up, professional help can aid ACoAs to see where and how different aspects of the illness impact on them. It strikes me, however, that one hour of therapy or 90 minutes of group therapy each week needs to be supplemented by two or three ACoA meetings weekly — especially during the early phase of recovery. For some ACoAs an hour of therapy barely scratches the surface of their issues.

ACoAs also need to be willing to form relationships with fellow ACoAs and to be in contact with them often. I firmly believe this. My fellow group members were my guides, showing me where and how I was in difficulty. I needed to open up to them many hours a week. I needed their companionship because I wanted to recover fully — something I could never accomplish alone.

CHAPTER 7

A Matter Of Faith

The Concept Of A Higher Power

As a spiritually based recovery program, ACoA asks its members to consider developing faith in a Higher Power, a spiritual force or truth of their understanding. No organized religion is involved in ACoA and no member is ever required to adopt any formal or even informal spiritual belief. The members of ACoA are merely asked to give consideration to a spiritual path, selecting whatever power or deity or cosmic force they feel comfortable with. For my own recovery I found a belief in a Spiritual Being to be healing and nurturing. I became willing to allow forces outside my control to aid in my recovery.

The concept of a Higher Power can be very disturbing for some people with an ACoA background. As children our authority figures were alcoholic or co-alcoholic parents who were emotionally distressed, and we received much abuse and betrayal from them. Consequently ACoAs find it very difficult to rely upon or have faith in any kind of power or central authority — even one of our own choosing. Our authority figures were threatening, dysfunctional parents who gave and withheld nurturing in an arbitrary and often cruel manner. Resistance is the most natural reaction in the world, to such experiences.

Many of us had tried to have faith in our parents with disastrous results. My own parents were extremely unpredictable. One day I would receive praise for something I did and the next day I would be rebuked for the same act. There was no consistency. I was alternately terrified and enraged at the authority figures in my childhood.

Coming to a receptive stance concerning the concept of a Higher Power in ACoA need not be painful, but it may involve considerable time. Fortunately most ACoAs I knew who were initially uncomfortable with or resisted a belief in a Higher Power eventually came to believe. Over time they embraced the concept of a power greater than themselves that could help them find a new understanding and self-acceptance. In the beginning I needed to suspend critical judgment about a Power greater than myself, to put my beliefs and considerations on the shelf. Then I began to listen to others and observe how they perceived their Higher Power. I never felt any pressure to believe in anything, only a suggestion that I set aside my long-standing perceptions and open myself up to the possibilities. And, like so many before me in other 12-Step programs, I did develop a belief in something beyond what I could directly see. I accepted that something was trying, lovingly, to guide both me and others. Slowly I gained conviction that some Higher Power was moving me toward wholeness and love. I could see this in my daily living. As I watched myself go through painful changes and achieve a kind of serenity I had never experienced, I began to see that I could not have done any of it alone.

Faith and spirituality are personal matters. It is difficult for people to articulate their personal beliefs in this area and it's even more difficult to describe in a book.

History is filled with events that have been attributed to faith in a Higher Power. The co-founders of the original 12-Step recovery program, Alcoholics Anonymous, stated very clearly that their strength and direction came from their faith in a Higher Power.

Agnostics and atheists as well as believers of all faiths are welcome in ACoA. We urge all who have grave reservations about faith in a Higher Power to momentarily set aside these considerations and just visit and experience the healing power of the ACoA meetings.

Those in ACoA who do have an abiding faith in a Higher Power have an additional source to draw upon. I know of no

more helpful path to healing and recovery than through a partnership effort with a Higher Power as you understand It. I
have, on many occasions, witnessed what I would describe as
miracles of faith. I have seen healing and growth where it
appeared to be all but impossible. I have seen joy and serenity
replace anguish and emotional disturbance. I have watched
ACoAs struggle with all manner of earthly problems and tri-
umph through faith. I firmly believe this faith and grace is
available to us all.

Prayer

Listening to other people proclaim how prayer has worked in
their lives doesn't bring me anywhere near the joy that comes
from actually experiencing responses to my own prayers. When
I pray, I feel as though I am having a conversation with my
Higher Power. In my conversations I generally ask for guidance
and direction. When I'm uncertain of which path to take, I ask
my Higher Power for love and understanding. Often I can readily see when I'm getting help. My mind will become quiet and
my thinking will gain clarity. Whenever fear or depression de-
scend on me with any intensity, I turn to the power of prayer to
carry me through.

When I can, I try to put myself in a quiet, contemplative
mood before I pray. I know that prayer doesn't require any
special environment, but I find that I become more focused and
centered when I get still.

Prayer doesn't work for me when I ask for things of this world
— money, a bigger car, fame, a new home or winning the lottery.
I suppose that if prayers in this realm were answered, I might
easily become distracted and use my energy for selfish pursuits.
And I've found that the longer I practice prayer (and meditation)
on a daily basis, the more I see it as a means of developing a
deeper spiritual bond with my Higher Power and a greater trust
and love for my fellow ACoA members. Prayer also puts me on
a journey to self-discovery. In my prayer I frequently ask to be
shown my motives, the nature of my pain and the true essence
of my fear or anger. This allows me to look behind the defenses
and screens I use to conceal myself from me.

I also find that prayer is extremely beneficial when I can't be
of direct help to someone in trouble or in need of support. I've

often implored my Higher Power, "Please help this person to do that which is healing and loving."

In all my activities I view prayer as a powerful tool for good. I suppose some members of ACoA might challenge my belief in prayer with an argument such as, "Prayers get answered only if you do the footwork." That may be part of the formula, or perhaps my Higher Power supplies both the motivation and the direction. I prefer to believe that my Higher Power also provides the energy I need to row the boat.

I'm certainly no miracle worker, but I have come to see some minor wonders accomplished. A prayer I use on a daily basis whenever I am in a fear-provoking situation is "Please, God, help me!" It helps to calm me. Prayer helps me achieve a connection with my Higher Power, and out of this I gain a renewed acceptance of myself. For many years I have struggled with the deprived lost child within me who resisted recovery. Prayer has been the principal tool I used to quiet him. My prayers for greater self-acceptance and self-knowledge carry me through some of my most difficult moments. And I know from talking with many hundreds of ACoA members that prayer has been equally helpful to them.

A curious thing about prayer is how seldom people discuss it. Whenever it is discussed, it's generally done with a degree of embarrassment or reticence. True, prayer is a very personal act; but I often wonder why grown men and women shy away from comment or discussion about such a powerful tool for recovery. These days I am only too willing to tell people about the role that prayer has played in my life and recovery.

Meditation

Years ago I was told that prayer was a way of talking to God and that meditation was an effective way of listening to God, and that the most effective form of prayer was deep listening. Since many people would rather do the talking than the listening, it's not surprising that meditation seems less popular than the prayer of petition. Some people are much more comfortable or secure when they are active. They have difficulty trying to sit quietly in a contemplative state. I think that the still, quiet voice of a Higher Power is more audible when the seeker is in a quiet meditative state. Unfortunately this world offers hundreds of distractions to keep us from this aspect of spiritual renewal.

For those who are not inclined to have faith in a Higher Power, meditation can be a wonderful way to reflect upon life, relationships and issues being confronted. Out of a still silence, understanding and answers can flow. Whatever their motives or beliefs, I suggest that all ACoAs make a consistent effort to engage in some form of meditation. My first experiences with it enabled me to quiet down my racing thoughts.

Meditation is the vehicle that enables me to have a richer spiritual life. I've tried to develop a special listening attitude. In meditation I open myself to instruction. I become truly willing and receptive, putting my wants and needs aside and adopting a posture of focused awareness and listening. I relax my body, concentrate on my breathing and do my best to become receptive. On occasion I will inhale "God," exhale "loves me." I do this to get calm and centered. It is when I'm calm and listening that I'm available for enlightenment and guidance.

I have also engaged in "light" meditation. In this effort I try to visualize light moving up my body in a healing manner.

I've described some of my approaches, but there are many forms of meditation available to the individual. The form you use is not nearly as important as your willingness to use meditation as a recovery tool. In my meditation efforts I try to make myself available to a Power greater than myself. I temporarily step out of the driver's seat to become teachable. By putting myself in a quiet listening mood I become open to direction however I may perceive it. I believe that deep listening is the highest form of love I can give to my Higher Power. Then I go about my life trying to be of service to myself and others.

In all of my meditative activities it's up to me to listen as intently as I can. When I let my mind wander to a wide range of topics, it's because I have lost my central focus. Concentration is sometimes difficult and my surroundings less than ideal, but with practice I have learned to tune out many distractions. It takes discipline to incorporate meditation into daily living, but you can engage in it anywhere, anytime. It's helpful if you can set aside a modest block of time — preferably at the same time each day — and adhere to this schedule as best you can until it becomes a familiar experience.

Resistance And Setbacks To Recovery

Recovery is a lifelong process. It cannot be accomplished overnight or by attendance at just a few meetings. I know, because as long and hard as I've been working on it, I am not "recovered." I experience recovery as an ongoing, upward spiral that provides greater depth of realization. So if you expect to accomplish recovery in a set amount of time, you may be sorely disappointed.

It requires a sustained effort to improve the quality of living and to build meaningful friendships with other group members. How members function in the ACoA group environment is a pretty clear representation of how they function in other areas of their life. It's difficult to be one kind of personality in ACoA and a distinctly different individual in other settings.

When an ACoA member is experiencing a great deal of resistance to recovery, it will probably show up in one or more of the following behavior patterns, most of which lead to a decrease in spontaneity and increased difficulty in trusting, sharing and feeling. All are pronounced signals of resistance and withdrawal.

Trying To Do It Alone

Often a newcomer will attend a few meetings, gather some information, make a rough assessment of the potential contribution of ACoA and then decide to work on his or her problems alone. It pains me when members of ACoA describe how their first approach to recovery was sidetracked by a decision to go it alone. An individual comes through the doors of ACoA; readily identifies with eight or nine issues in the Laundry List; completely relates to much of the sharing by members—and then decides to try the "home-study" method of recovery. Such activity is self-defeating.

It's a tragic mistake for newcomers to turn their back on any recovery program that speaks directly to so many personal problems. And yet this happens every day all over the world. The "I can do it myself" approach, which was probably an early survival mode, shuts off so many people from a healthy new way of living. Like most ACoAs, I need human beings in my life to help me recover. I had to surrender my isolated pose of self-reliance. I needed to share, to trust others, to identify and to feel. I learned about my disease through others and in partnership with them. I cannot recover alone and I don't know many people who can.

Trying to change in isolation is far too limiting. Life is all about relationships. And if I'm having problems with relationships—and I think most ACoAs do—then I have to work them through by learning about my actions, my contributions to the problems. I can only do this with the feedback and insight provided by other people, and readily available to me in the ACoA recovery program.

A Sometime Thing

Those in AA often quote the wonderful phrase "Half-measures availed us nothing." It aptly refers to the degree of willingness and commitment of the individual seeking recovery. Too often the newcomer makes the judgment that he or she can "audit" the course—just sit in for a quick refresher.

Believe me when I say that I wish ACoA could be used in such a progressive manner. In reality, however, members grow and change and recover because they are ready and willing to show up regularly and do the hard work.

Sitting on the fence doesn't work. Such troublesome issues as extensive people-pleasing, fear of abandonment, over-responsibility and stuffing of feelings seldom respond favorably to half-measures. Once an individual has accepted the fact that they do, indeed, have some real behavior problems that can be attributed to an alcoholic upbringing, only a committed and sustained effort can bring solid relief. Anything less is just a form of evasion.

Recovery takes time, effort and a willingness to learn about feelings, a desire to experience good and bad feelings and a readiness to risk telling others. In ACoA we concentrate on feelings—depressing ones, uncomfortable ones, frightening ones. We try to experience and re-experience painful moments in a safe, supportive environment. A person who is just passing through probably will not sit still or pay attention long enough to reap any substantial benefits from these efforts.

Haphazard attendance is one way to stay isolated and apart from the group. In all probability the members of the group will adopt a casual, distant attitude toward the individual just as the individual has with them. This is very self-defeating.

Wanting A Quick Fix

As children we saw our parents do many patch-up jobs to the family problems. And we were probably served many quick-fix TV dinners and remedies for minor colds—overnight relief from pain and suffering. It seemed to work well for a while, but eventually things broke down worse than before.

The quick solution is seldom an enduring one. Nonetheless many ACoAs still try to get by with a series of magical fixes.

I'm pretty much like everyone else, and I definitely hoped for a quick magical cure — a high-intensity resolution to all my problems. When I first began in ACoA I was willing to put out some effort but I wanted fast response, quick recovery. In short, I had high expectations. I was almost childlike in my expectations that our fledgling ACoA program would provide fast, fast relief for my symptoms!

I gambled a lot as a young man. With gambling there's a short time between the bet and the results, and I grew accustomed to fast results. As a stockbroker I bought and sold stocks for myself and my clients. If I didn't see immediately favorable results, I moved the investments elsewhere. I brought this same mentality with me to early ACoA. I was hoping for the ultimate quick fix—a short trip from turmoil to emotional well-being.

Well, it didn't work for me and I seriously doubt that it can work for anyone else. Recovery turned out to be a lot of hard work. My really deep-rooted issues did not readily yield to my new insights. It took new behavior and new attitudes to begin to heal them — neither of which I was able to acquire in a few months. If my experience is at all representative, then I would suggest that newcomers gently let go of any dreams of a quick fix and settle in for the real miracles.

Unwillingness To Share And Open Up

Just listening to others and reading the literature—trying to get well just through gathering information—probably won't produce many positive results. An important element in ACoA recovery is self-disclosure—a willingness to tell the group as a whole, and selected individuals, what is really going on in one's life. I need to share my feelings about my problems. The reality is, I have all these problems. It's a "feeling illness" that I'm grappling with and it can't be resolved with knowledge alone.

One of the most threatening aspects of the ACoA recovery program is the intense, revelatory level of sharing. Long-buried shame, confusion and rage surface and all the pain and anguish that go with them are shared. Twelve-Step recovery programs succeed because the members are willing to open up to fellow members, become human and vulnerable. All of this is doubly necessary in ACoA because it is such a devastating and all-encompassing feeling disease.

Newcomers in ACoA soon see the value and merit of sharing. It is a release, a relief and it signifies a willingness to let go and feel the feelings. Unfortunately some members are so rigid and intimidated by the meetings and the recovery process that they remain silent and withdrawn. True, some meetings can be intense and on occasion full of anger. But there is no way that a member can benefit from a sphinx-like demeanor. There may be great silent heroes in the movies; but in ACoA those who cloak themselves in silence, seriously limit their recovery prospects. Self-acceptance and self-love come out of sharing and owning who you are. We generally loathe our hidden self and self-loathing, shame and evasion form a pattern that ACoA recovery hopes to reverse.

Opening up to people can be frightening. It involves risk, rejection and criticism. In ACoA, however, judgment and criticism are almost nonexistent. There may be some low-level gossip and a few personality clashes but the overall environment is supportive, noncritical and noninvasive. This is the only way that ACoA can adequately function as a recovery program.

We are brought together to share as brothers and sisters, to heal each other. This is something we cannot do alone or in silence. We can trust the process, surrender to it and try not to retreat into silence. I never could think my way out of my problems. I had to feel, act and talk my way out of them. Quite often the ACoA program asks people to do that which they fear and hate as part of the recovery — and it works.

Drifting And Not Focusing On Personal Problems

Newcomers to ACoA are shown a list of behavior patterns that have brought problems and troubles to all of us. As newcomers listen to members share, they discover other characteristics and issues.

Most members readily identify with some of the major issues and add to their "to be worked on" list as they make progress in their recovery. Some members, however, seem to have difficulty identifying just what it is they should be working on. They are vague and unfocused. They may be able to share at great length about how much they were abused as children, but often they don't see clearly that it's all connected to their current behavior. They need to sit quietly and draw up their very own list of problems. They can either focus on the most troublesome ones, or attack the least difficult ones if they have trouble confronting and working on some of the larger issues.

Another way to limit recovery is to just drift along without understanding that recovery requires work. It's sad to watch members drift like leaves on a windy pond, moved around by forces outside themselves. To ignore one's issues is to ignore the program. The program can always provide some nourishment to the drifters but real change and progress will probably elude them until they define and take responsibility for their problems with a concerted effort.

My own self-deception was a major hindrance to my recovery. Since I had written the Laundry List and thrown myself into service, helping to put the groups on solid footing, I felt that I was doing wonders with my own ACoA illness. But after a few years I realized that I had blithely skipped over some of my issues — I hadn't done the core work that was required. Because I was the originator of the Laundry List, I had deceived myself into thinking I had cleaned up some problems when all I had done was define them and give them lip service.

In ACoA there is an essential process that cannot be avoided. Members have to prepare their own precise list of issues. Then they need to develop some recovery goals, specifying what they want to accomplish and how they will proceed. Remember, your Higher Power will steer you, but you need to do the rowing.

Avoiding The ACoA 12 Steps Of Recovery

Sometimes members can get so carried away with the dynamics of the sharing process and the recitation of their problems that they ignore the important framework that holds the ACoA structure together: the ACoA 12 Steps. These steps are meant to be incorporated into daily life.

The central themes of the steps focus on love and understanding. We are asked to undertake the task of reversing our behavior and start loving ourselves. To do this requires a certain amount of surrender, some examination of our parents and ourselves and a willingness to correct wrongs and grow along spiritual lines.

Working most steps is a solitary affair. Some members prefer the excitement and challenges of the meetings and social fellowship to the singular process of step work. Yet it is essential that we keep the focus on ourselves. The steps help make this possible.

The ACoA 12 Steps offer nourishment, not punishment. ACoAs have had enough punishment in their lives. The steps accelerate self-awareness, and for many they will be the first real opportunity to develop a relationship with a Higher Power.

Despite all these benefits some members may not actively work the steps. Others may jump in only to fade when they arrive at steps four and five. Some may resist undertaking an inventory of their parents. Perhaps they will feel that such actions are betrayal of the family secrets or maybe they prefer to bury the past.

Many members are disturbed when they see that they have many of the same behavior patterns as their dysfunctional parents. This is simply a fact. Our early training system was our parents, and we invariably learned to respond to life in much the same way as our parents. Blame is not an issue; we are merely trying to examine the dimensions of the problem behavior and be aware of its influence and the impact of it on our lives.

Perfectionism

The desire to be perfect in performance, knowledge or behavior is a perplexing character trait that definitely works against recovery. I believe that perfectionism is created by fear. This was certainly true for me. I became a perfectionist because I was afraid of punishment. If I didn't do something perfectly I might be rejected, ridiculed, fired, abandoned or ignored. Many people become perfectionists to please the world. My ACoA issue involving perfectionism also stems from an effort to control the outside world so that I won't be hurt but will be accepted and loved. So my efforts at perfection were aimed at favorably influencing what I perceived to be a hostile, unfriendly world.

In ACoA we ask people to turn inward, to respect the inner self and not stay stuck in pleasing the external world. Perfectionism involves greater effort and energy, much of which could be rechanneled to a sensible application of program principles.

Such suggestions as "Easy does it—but do it," "Lower your standards and your performance will rise" and "Think" can help the perfectionist to loosen the grip of fear. Overly responsible individuals are particularly troubled by perfectionism in all sorts of matters. Fortunately there is no possibility of working the ACoA program perfectly! How well we work the program will be reflected in how we feel about ourselves and in the nature of our relationship with our Higher Power. Only we can judge the results.

Instant Relationships

Developing friendships with members of your ACoA groups is a healthy activity. It demonstrates a willingness to reach out, open up and share. There is, however, one social approach that can be troublesome, especially for those in the first year of recovery.

Too often newcomers become prematurely involved with ACoA members of the opposite sex. They form instant physical relationships with each other. This is natural — common issues and a sense of family tend to draw people together. Sometimes it is a lost child calling to a rescuer. Instant romance however, takes a great deal of time, attention and energy. The new romantic has shifted his or her center away from recovery to the demands of the new relationship. And sadly, I know of no self-help recovery program that can compete with a new romance. Thus it generally leads to a setback or slowdown in the recovery process.

The "me" that first shows up at an ACoA meeting is usually quite desperate and emotionally troubled in the area of relationships. The newcomer is often very needy and confused. Many members of ACoA endorse the concept of focusing solely on yourself if you arrived at ACoA unattached. The operating principle for this suggestion is that there has got to be a solid "me" before there can be an "us." Common sense points to waiting until you are more secure in the knowledge of who you are. It's best to view group activity as an opportunity for awareness and growth rather than romance. And, since the group can take on the characteristics of the family of origin, ill-conceived romantic endeavors with other group members can tear apart the new healthy family concept.

In a new romantic involvement it is most common for ACoAs to act out the old dramas of earlier attachments. ACoA newcomers need time to see the nature and complexity of their relationship issues. Involvement in a romance with another ACoA — especially another newcomer — can only serve to short-circuit recovery and possibly drive the newcomer away from the program. The focus needs to be on personal recovery not on a romantic conquest. Unfortunately many ACoAs are just awakening to incest issues and trying to resolve them. In their efforts to grow and recreate their early family, physical attachments and involvements can be very damaging. The best suggestion I can give is to take it easy and remember that recovery needs to come first.

Fixing Others

I'm never sure where the boundary between sharing and rescuing is located. For some members of ACoA, giving advice and fixing others is as natural as breathing. As young children in an alcoholic household, their assigned role was one of rescuer, fixer and hero. The actions of a fixer generally go far beyond general support and sharing. Fixers attach themselves to other members and often attempt to run their lives, professing to have most of the answers to whatever problems the "victim" is facing. Fixing others gives stature, importance and control to an individual — three good reasons to engage in it.

A somewhat less intrusive form of fixing is chronic advice-giving. Most meetings have one or two "senior advisers" who feel it is their mission to dispense advice — not share experiences in a give-and-take manner — to the more confused, suffering members of the group.

I think we can draw a distinction between fixing, advising and sharing. The first two are intrusive and involve giving up one's center. Sharing is a different mechanism. Ideally, sharing involves relating one's experiences, perhaps how a person handled a particularly troubling issue. It is done in a passive, nondirective manner: "If you can benefit from my experiences, please do. If not, that's okay."

Fixing and advising can seriously interfere with recovery of both the fixer and the person being fixed. The fixer is often acting out of a need to stay away from his or her problems — helping others is a sure way to avoid personal issues. Fixing also has a component of control to it, an issue many ACoAs are trying to resolve. It's commendable to want to steer others through tough times that you have experienced and resolved. But if it interferes with your own growth (and it usually does) or that of the newcomer, it's best to step aside. We are in ACoA to fix ourselves, not others.

In those situations where a formal sponsor-sponsee relationship is in place, both parties agree that mutual *sharing* and *exploration* of problems will characterize the relationship. In this arrangement guidance is best given when it is open to change or reversal. The demanding, overbearing, controlling sponsor can do the sponsee a real disservice. Unfortunately some newcomers are drawn to strong, directive personalities because that's the kind of individual who ran their childhood home. Early ACoA linkages are often based upon old family dynamics. This recreation of early family roles in ACoA is inevitable but sometimes troubling.

In my alcoholic household I was always preoccupied with the feelings of my parents. When they felt gloomy, I felt gloomy and threatened. I wanted people close to me to feel good so I could feel good. In ACoA I had to learn to let others feel troubled, depressed, miserable, lost or fearful without rushing over and trying to fix them. I learned to detach and not pick up and carry another's burden. Trying to fix others is a selfish, time-consuming way of continuing to feed my illness.

Denial And Blame

It's still very easy for me to be blind to the essence of some of my actions. There are issues in my life that don't yield easily to clarity. I literally can't see the forest for the trees. Sometimes I finally reach discovery and understanding on my own. More often, however, the insight and inspiration comes from someone sharing at a meeting, or my observation of another member's blindness.

This is why meetings and friendships in ACoA can be so meaningful. Where I have been absolutely blind to a destructive trait for many years — let's say arrogance, a controlling nature or vicious gossiping — it's not very likely that I will quickly single it out and resolve it in ACoA. I may have to see it in others or feel the resistance of others to my negative actions.

Even more helpful is a loving sponsor who gently points to some of my blind spots and eases me into a recognition of how I have been hurting myself. Denial is the mind's way of defending itself from fear, feelings of inadequacy and a whole legion of hurts. Left alone, denial can make a real mess of recovery. A willingness to examine one's actions, to be open to feedback from others and to seek the aid of a sponsor or close friend in ACoA can shorten the distance between blindness and discovery.

Blaming others is a natural way to shift attention away from the responsibility to recover. For example, if I spend all my emotional energy blaming my parents for the issues that are repeatedly troubling me I stay blind to the need to engage in my own recovery. Blame is corrosive; it blinds and enables one to remain free from responsible actions. Yes, it's true our parents taught us miserably, if they taught us at all. But recovery will come when we admit to ourselves and others how enraged, hurt and helpless we have always felt about them. Then we can experience it all and move on to positive change.

Does The ACoA Recovery Program Work?

CHAPTER 9

Can I Really Change?

Recovery is not an easy process. For the newcomer full of hope, recovery and change may appear to be the automatic dividends of regular attendance, devotion to the program and spiritual development. Nice as this would be, it's just not true.

I view recovery as lying along a spectrum. At one end is "virtually no change" and at the other end is "deep substantive change." The entire spectrum is available through the ACoA program.

Some members won't stay active and committed long enough to make more than limited progress on the journey. I have known others who persevered and did achieve remarkable emotional well-being. These winners understood at a deep level that they were sick and tired of living a tolerable half-life. They came to a point where they were willing to go to any length to bring about true substantive change in their behavior and their relationships with others.

That any ACoA can change is a given. As soon as someone walks through the doors of an ACoA meeting, hears and identifies with the Laundry List and the personal sharing of the members, the process of change has begun. When the individual

begins to understand the nature of the problems and how childhood disturbances created chronic and continuing problems,
the journey truly begins. The extent of change depends on the
ACoA's willingness to continue the journey.

So the answer to the question is, "Yes, anyone can change,
and for some this change can be deep and formidable." The
extensive changes that I have seen and experienced cover a
wide range of issues. Whether it was a problem with abandonment, fear of authority figures, guilt, control or inability to
express stuffed feelings, healing change took place after a concerted effort in recovery. Change is probably most evident in
the meetings.

Over time I have watched suspicious, angry and rigid members become open, accepting and trusting. This to me was trans-
formation of the most fundamental kind. I have also observed
desperately shy and frightened, dependent individuals emerge
from their constricted world and become confident, independent
and whole.

Over the years I've had a real opportunity in ACoA to witness many miracles. What saddens me most are those who start
the journey only to fade and retreat once again into denial after
just three or four meetings. I have to keep remembering that
they are not at fault. It is their disease that diverts them from
a chance to bring about true, wholesome change in their lives.
For those who persevere, the rewards are many.

When I am asked how long it will take for substantive change
to occur, I can only share that each person's recovery is different.
No two people will grow and change at the same rate. I do
know, however, that the more effort, the more attention paid to
issues, the more risking in new areas, the better the chances are
for an early recovery from some difficult problems. I can't stress
enough how much hard work is required in order to achieve
long-lasting change.

Surface or cosmetic change is relatively easy; ACoAs do it all
the time. A little knowledge and sharing can sometimes mislead
newcomers into believing they have made great strides — until
they collide with some of their more enduring and resistant
patterns of behavior. For all ACoAs it's very discouraging and
humbling to discover that an issue you thought you had overcome was right back causing great difficulty. I counsel newcomers not to expect immediate recovery in such areas as control,
fear and rage. Little issues and problems yield more readily.

Some issues and behavior patterns will require long-term alertness. For everyone, ACoA or not, old habit pattterns die hard. It's up to us to outlast their influence upon us.

In ACoA change comes from being willing to alter our reactions as well as our actions. I had to learn not to react to the sickness in others. I taught myself not to overreact to strong or rude criticism. I had to slow down and examine my reactions to outside stimuli. At parties, in money matters, with my children, I had to get past old automatic responses (most of which were fear-based) and give myself time to think. I also had to stop all of my violent critical attacks on myself. This latter problem I changed by using positive affirmations and visualizations to replace my scathing denunciations when I acted inappropriately or blundered in some way. Over and over I would say to myself, "I love you, Tony. You did the best you could."

The whole ACoA process is one of change. People come through the doors with some incredibly destructive beliefs and behavior patterns. The task of ACoA is to enable and guide people through some much-needed change. The fact that there are meetings and people sitting together sharing about their problems, drawing strength from each other, trusting, feeling and revealing who they really are is a clear indication to me that ACoA can bring real change to its members.

What Is Recovery?

Every ACoA's perception of recovery is different. No two individuals will have the same impressions and expectations. One may be looking forward to a new spontaneity and truly satisfying relationships, while another may be seeking a peaceful serenity with an end to anxiety and fear. In truth, recovery can be all of these and much more.

Any effort to portray recovery needs to focus on the most common patterns at the core of our being. Like all other ACoAs, my recovery efforts have been aimed at surrendering and letting go of a whole series of inappropriate defenses. At the same time I am actively developing a blameless understanding of myself and taking positive actions that I know can lead to self-acceptance and self-love. For years I lived a life of shame, secrecy and desperation and I yearned for an existence where I could be at peace with myself and others — a state that's not easy to attain in today's stress-filled world.

Regardless of our denial or our successes in life, I think that most unrecovering ACoAs are painfully aware that they are not functioning well. They sense that something is terribly amiss. Unfortunately they join most of their neighbors in the great conspiracy called, "Let's keep our pain and our humanity concealed." Everyone gets to play this game of "act as if." Some do it well; others have little capacity for it and seek help; still others get addicted and go crazy. It takes real courage to enter a self-help recovery program such as ACoA. And it takes even greater valor to start revealing the long-hidden family secrets and our continued sick responses to them.

Recovery is a wondrous, inspired, ongoing process. Newcomers walk through the doors of ACoA barely able to articulate the nature and substance of the pain that brought them to the meeting. They can only say, "I don't want to be this way any longer." They actually are willing to surrender the very defenses and behavior patterns that helped them survive in their alcoholic household. They begin the awesome process of changing their lifelong reponses and actions. With the help of others and a Higher Power, their sick, distorted thinking begins to heal and they start to feel the gift of emotional wellbeing. This gift is something they will have to nurture and tend to for the rest of their lives, but it is a task that becomes easier as self-love blossoms.

Recovery is . . .

- An expanding process of self-understanding
- Creating and sustaining supportive, mutually enjoyable personal relationships
- Having the ability to feel and experience a full range of emotions in wholesome and appropriate ways
- Being clear about one's needs and being able to ask to have them met in a positive manner
- Taking healthy actions and risks that will lead to increased self-acceptance
- Confronting problems and difficulties with confidence in an ability to resolve them effectively

- A willingness to grow along spiritual lines
- Emotional balance and a state of well-being.

Being A Healthy Parent
To Our Wounded Child Within

In our first few years upon this earth we had an opportunity to be vital, spontaneous human beings, full of hope and confidence. But something happened — and the sick family environment put an end to our infant chances for a wholesome upbringing. Instead our infant was neglected or abused for many years, without hope, without healthy nurture and above all without understanding.

In adult life many former infants try to heal their abandoned child by "doing," by compensating for the sense of shame and worthlessness that they carry with them. The greater the outer display, the greater the inner poverty. Finally, with the help of ACoA, we began to understand that healing could only be realized by going within and rescuing the abandoned child. In order to heal the pain we were asked to embrace it, feel it, sit quietly and re-experience all the hurt, torment, abuse and helplessness. We were told that such actions could bring our child into the light. For many it took an incredible act of faith to bridge a lifetime of emotional defenses and begin rescue efforts. Once the abandoned child has been brought into the light, nurturing is essential to keep it from slipping back into the darkness once again.

Each of us needs to learn how to give nourishment to that part of ourselves that has been locked away for so long. The child is the core spirit that we carry. That spirit needs to be acknowledged, accepted and loved. In my journey I turned to affirmations each day. The first day I began saying, "I love you little Tony." I was embarrassed and wanted to run. Slowly, however, I began to get a new sense of myself. I also used visualizations. I would create a mind picture of the adult me hugging and protecting the abandoned infant me. I formed a relationship with this other me. I made it a sacred and cherished one. I knew that I had to develop a loving acceptance of this other me and that my loathing and self-hatred were all inside this lost child. Over time I fully adopted this child and became a responsible, caring parent.

I realize that the foregoing passages might leave you wondering about my sanity! Let me say that just as I believe that I have a Higher Power to call on for help, I also believe that there is a lost little child in me at the core of my being. I think that life became so painful for that child that it licked its wounds and went off to a dark corner. This child needed to be acknowledged. I needed to re-experience all of this lost child's hurt and shame, own it and free the child. Deep inside I knew that until I liberated this child and nurtured it, I couldn't be fully integrated.

CHAPTER 10

What To Do
About Parents

The Family Soap Opera

Early in childhood our parents assigned us a role in the family soap opera. We had no choice about the part we were directed to play, and we were never allowed the right to reject the role if it didn't seem to fit or was downright destructive. We were in a helpless position: We had no say about our immediate destiny.

As the illness in the household grew it expanded and disabled everyone. As helpless children we took on the characteristics of the disease. Out of necessity and a desire to survive we made adjustments to the family drama. We began to experience guilt and shame about the family illness. We were victimized on a daily basis with physical or verbal abuse, unwarranted and inconsistent punishment and a litany of hundreds of critical observations such as "Shame on you," "How can we love anyone who does that," "You'll just drive your father to drink if you do that," "God won't love you if . . . ," "You shouldn't feel that way."

As children we were absolutely unable to see what was really going on. We couldn't see that we were in no way responsible for our parents' drinking or other destructive behavior. The responsibility rested squarely with them. We didn't cause their alcoholism, we couldn't control it (God knows, we tried!), and we certainly couldn't cure it. In all probability their sick and

99

distorted reactions to life came directly out of their own painful, distressing upbringing. They too were victims. They were merely passing along their sick heritage. In the family dynamic the whole family enables and covers for the alcoholic in hopes that they will change. Eventually many ACoAs shut down, detach and accept at the core of their being that they were the cause or contributing cause of the family illness.

In ACoA I had to get very clear that I didn't cause my father's rage just because I had an accident in the bathroom. And I didn't cause my mother to die by being a "bad boy." I was innocent on all counts, but back then I believed at the core of my soul that I was the cause. Today I have to be ever alert lest I inappropriately accept blame or guilt.

As an adult in ACoA I can change my early script. First I need awareness, to understand that the role I played as a child for my parents' benefit was a sick one. And, if I continue to play that role and repeat those actions as an adult, it will only make me sicker. I must fully accept without reservation that I did not cause my parents to drink. As a little child I didn't have that kind of power, though many times I wished I had the power to stop their insane behavior.

Our Personal Rage And Sorrow

Two very powerful emotions buffet the ACoA about: an emerging rage at one's parents and a deep, aching sorrow over a lost childhood. Alcohol and the family environment that went with it robs all ACoAs of a healthy, spontaneous and nurturing childhood. Our youthful joys were always being trampled by the family sickness. For most of us one of the truly damaging aspects of being raised in an alcoholic household was our treatment as a nonperson. Part of this process of being robbed of any individuality as a human being was the need to stuff feelings of anger and resistance. In my family there was only one person who could directly express anger and rage: my father. The rest of us had to suppress our anger at how we were treated. We were not valued, and this was never more evident than in the way our feelings and needs were so conveniently ignored. Year after year I was forced to stuff my feelings until somewhere deep inside me I developed this molten ball of rage at all the times I had been abused and invalidated.

I think that this core of rage is within all ACoAs and all abused children. Many ACoAs have shared how their rage became strangled by their loyalty to their parents. How could parents be wrong? Parents were to be respected — not because of what they did and how they treated us but just because they were our parents. Therefore we must be mistaken in our perceptions of them. Always, it seems we were the ones who were wrong, inappropriate, stupid and foolish.

Just how the ball of rage was created varies from person to person. But for just about every one of us it is there and we need to deal with it in recovery.

Suggestions For Healing

Where our parents are concerned, popular opinion might easily take us down a path that has only two recovery steps: awareness and forgiveness. Time and again, however, ACoAs have shared how this particular approach didn't work for them. The cumulative rage had stayed stuffed. The grieving over the lost childhood had been dismissed as self-indulgent or theatrical.

Theory has it that once you are aware of the real nature of a situation (our parents' alcoholism), you are then able to move on to forgiving them their disease, as they too were victims. But ACoA suggests that there is a central issue that absolutely needs to be addressed before a person can reach the forgiveness stage. We cannot rationalize or intellectualize our way through this stage, we have to experience it in all its intensity. That immense well of rage and self-pity needs to be brought to the surface and openly experienced. Until this is done, dealing with parents is largely an exercise in futility.

We absolutely need to feel all those mind-numbing feelings of helplessness and the rage it triggered then and will trigger now as we relive those distant days. It can't remain blocked. It's a poison in our system and it needs to be brought up if we are to recover. Most ACoAs need to feel the rage and sorrow over and over again until it is spent. This generally can't be achieved in a single week. Believe me when I say that all ACoAs have a huge reservoir of pain to contend with, not a neat, tidy thimbleful.

Finding a safe outlet for all this pent-up, suppressed bile is essential. Many of us have spent our adult years venting this rage at inappropriate times, directing it at those who resembled or represented our parents. Most likely the sorrow has made us distant, unavailable and depressed. We were experiencing minor volcanic eruptions, and some of the lava was getting to the surface where it singed friends, spouse and children but seldom, if ever, our alcoholic parents.

ACoA meetings offer a safe, secure, supportive environment where we can begin to experience these powerful feelings and express them. ACoA members understand what is happening and do not invalidate the member who has just gotten in touch with a core of pure rage. Sometimes when members erupt, it can be frightening and uncomfortable. Some new members become very disturbed by the process and retreat. It's amazing how at a funeral relatives are encouraged to wail and get in touch with their grief and sorrow; experience it fully right at the grave site; exhaust themselves over many hours and days of active mourning. This process is seen as restorative and wholesome. In ACoA expressing rage and sorrow at one's parents and what happened in our childhood is equally restorative. It's a rite of passage to a new life. Don't be afraid of the process. Encourage it in yourself and in others. Try to be considerate of others when you express your rage but, more importantly, don't supress or cut off the rage and sorrow.

Some of us work with our rage in the following ways:

- Share with one or two close friends in a safe location and shout out what you feel.
- At home, hit pillows, cushions or a punching bag to absorb the energy that goes with your fury, accompanied by all the words you never expressed.
- Go into the woods and scream at the universe, your Higher Power or whatever representation fits. If you live near a beach, you can yell at the top of your voice at the surf.
- Write a letter to parents without editing or toning down your passion and rage. Then read it over a few times and share it with a supportive and understanding friend. But don't mail it!

If you're confronting sorrow, write about the broken promises and the hurt of the lost child within you. Describe all those moments that failed. Most ACoAs will confirm that holding onto these powerful emotions eventually will cause some kind of illness, either physical or emotional. The human body often produces a stress-related illness that reflects the pain and rage being stuffed.

Confronting Our Parents

Some ACoAs feel that it is essential that they communicate their feelings to their parents. If your parents are alive you can write them, telephone them or visit them. If your parent(s) are deceased you always can ask a supportive friend to play their silent role while you unburden yourself.

In any direct sharing with your parents there are some risks:

- Parents' denial that there was alcoholism or sick behavior.
- Debate about the severity of the problems.
- Outright attack, criticism and invalidation of what you say and who you are.
- Indifference and remoteness.
- Belief that the children or outside circumstances caused all of the problems.

When you approach your parents directly, it's best to keep in mind that they . . .

- Probably won't agree with your interpretations and views of what happened.
- Probably won't react as you would like — that is, admitting to it all, apologizing and begging for forgiveness.
- Probably won't change their way of treating you to any extent. Your role and their way of treating you was established many years ago.
- May decide to punish you in some way for bringing up old pain. They may even cease contact with you.

Many confrontations lead to a sort of touchy and suspicious armistice. Clear-cut victory is rare. It goes against human nature. Often what the ACoA really desires is that the parents suddenly transform themselves into the loving, nurturing, sensitive parents they just couldn't be because of their illness. This set of events will require understanding and acceptance on the part of the ACoA. The only element of the family soap opera we can change is who we are and how we choose to behave. A forthright and direct approach to our parents can, however, lead to a new and more meaningful relationship. We can establish a more honest, fearless level of communication. A new sense of respect and understanding can emerge out of confrontation. Such actions can be freeing as long as we don't have unreasonable expectations concerning the outcome. In short we can decide to accept our parents even if they make no changes or adjustments.

Leaving Home Emotionally

We start to leave home emotionally when we stop reacting negatively to some of the situations and people our parents and family always reacted to. When we can act spontaneously and responsibly in familiar stressful situations that created chaos in our family, then we have successfully begun our emotional journey away from our parents.

Unconsciously many of us stay tied to toxic parents much longer than we know. I'm reminded of one group member who spent months lamenting the fact that she was, for economic reasons, still living with her abusive mother. Finally she informed us that she had moved out and taken her own apartment. Six months later we discovered that her new apartment was located directly below her mother's in the same building.

The ties that bind can be truly powerful. There are many ways to stay unhealthily linked to your parents in a dependent and leaning manner:

- Living with parent(s) in their home.
- Being fully or partially supported (financially) by one or both parents.
- Spending most or all of your spare time with your parents rather than developing friendships with contemporaries and peers.
- Always vacationing with parents.
- Fully or partially supporting parents out of feelings of guilt or obligation.
- Daily visits, daily phone calls, working for parents' company are all ways to keep the old dynamics fresh.

Keep in mind that in the above scenarios the important factor is that our parent(s) continue to treat us in destructive, punishing or indifferent ways that are similar in manner to our childhood treatment and evoke the same kinds of negative responses. We are still buried alive. In our dealings with our parents we continue to lose our spontaneity, our aliveness — our independent selves. Some of us need to stay clear of toxic parents during early recovery.

Once an individual has embraced ACoA and come to understand the nature of the illness, stress and conflict with parents (especially those who are still alcoholically active) is quite natural. The family secrets are no longer sacred. We stop making excuses for our parents' sick behavior. We also may learn how we enable parents to continue their toxic journey. We resist and eventually repudiate the guilty, overresponsible victim role.

As we detach emotionally, our parents and their injunctions no longer control us. It is at this point that conflict becomes most intense. As we declare ourselves to be worthwhile, valued human beings who deserve respect, our sickness abates but not necessarily that of our parents. This leaves a void that needs special attention. At this juncture we can begin to address the issue of forgiveness.

Forgiving Our Parents

Of all the tasks we are asked to consider in ACoA, none is more challenging than a willingness to forgive. Forgiveness and letting go of judgments about our parents is a major point of recovery. We need to be responsible for the way in which we hold or cherish our parents.

Before we can move into this critical arena, before we can do healing work with our parents, there is one prerequisite: forgiveness of self. In order to forgive my parents I had to start by forgiving myself. I had to travel well down the action road to personal recovery. Forgiving myself meant that I had developed a new and positive understanding of myself. I accepted that I was a valuable and lovable human being and I took actions, daily, to reinforce that belief. My faith in myself had to be matched by actions. Once I reached this stage in forgiving myself I could begin the task of forgiving my parents. The logic is as follows:

- I unwittingly took on most of the characteristics of both my parents.
- These behavior patterns and beliefs are all inside me.
- The traits I most disliked in them, I carry.

- I must accept, embrace and work at changing these negative traits in me.
- Once I have neutralized them in me I can move on to forgiving my parents for these traits and how they harmed me.
- It's difficult to forgive my parents' behavior if I loathe or deny that same behavior in myself.

I may have traveled an entirely different road in my life and made every effort not to be like my parents, but I am. And as I work the fourth step of ACoA recovery and undertake a blameless review of my parents' behavior patterns, I will come face to face with my own defects and shortcomings. I must see that in stressful situations I typically recreated the dysfunctional behavior of my parents. As a child I had no choice. Their sickness was my model, my teaching system. As I work on myself to change these destructive patterns, I am laying the groundwork for forgiving my parents.

Now comes the most difficult part of the effort to forgive your parents — and for many it is a monumental effort. Here spirituality and compassion combine to produce a willingness to honestly contemplate and work along a forgiveness path. This path might consist of the following guidelines:

- Develop an understanding of the handicapped or desperate family environment your parents came from. Their sick survival mechanisms were the best they could do with what they inherited from their family environment.
- Visualize, if you can, your parents as frightened, abused children, trying to escape and surivive the insanity of their early households.
- Use prayer and meditation to help you understand that your parents did the best they could. Try to see that they could barely be there for themselves because they too were childhood victims.
- Accept the fact that your parents had or still have an illness that distorts and destroys life's joys. They are alcoholics, co-alcoholics or para-alcoholics.
- Acknowledge that at the present time their way of dealing with their actions and attitudes toward you may consist of denial, resistance or indifference.

- Pray for a continued willingness to let go of your judgments about them and to gain a recognition that if there is a culprit, it is the disease of alcoholism and the ways in which it ravaged your parents.

This process helps us to move toward an acceptance of our parents' humanity just as we have opened up to our own humanity and that of our fellow ACoA members.

Every ACoA needs to understand that forgiveness of one's parents is a way to increase one's valuation of oneself. It is a critical element in your healing process. By working on this element we are choosing to move away from hatred, retaliation, blame, judgment and scorn — a group of traits that can only diminish our efforts to achieve self-love.

The Individual And The Group: Some Lessons Learned

CHAPTER 11

Group Conscience

Like all 12-Step recovery programs, ACoA strives to adopt a democratic process. The individual is all important. The program is structured so that each member has a vote regarding matters that affect the group as a whole. The newcomer has a single vote, as does the old-timer with many years of group attendance. Moreover, any group member has a right to petition the chairman for a group vote. That is, an expression of group consciousness concerning any matter involving the ACoA group. To be effective, this vote is absolutely binding.

Votes are typically taken concerning such issues as election of group leaders, affiliation with a national organization, meeting hours, disbursement of group treasury funds to the host facility (church, school and so on) and purchase of literature. Groups also may vote on the type of meeting to be held: open (to the public) or closed (for Adult Children of Alcoholics only, not for those with other types of parental issues). Some meetings are composed solely of members of AA, and these are closed to all who are not members of AA. By and large, however, most ACoA meetings are open to the public at large.

109

My hope has always been that each group should build their doors as wide as possible to accommodate those who came from a wide variety of dysfunctional backgrounds. All indications are that we ACoAs are not particularly different in our reactions to a sick family than those who came from a dysfunctional home where a compulsion such as drugs, gambling or sexual abuse was the root of the illness.

In an ACoA group, the leaders need to remember that they are but trusted servants, not masters of the castle. Sensitivity to the needs and desires of others is a most helpful quality. Autocratic rule is very unpopular at ACoA meetings and is to be discouraged.

Groups usually hold elections every six months and elect a new slate of officers. Everyone is encouraged to participate, especially those who are shy and uncomfortable with the group.

Usually a business meeting is held for the purpose of holding elections and discussing group matters. Since most of us came from homes ruled by dictators or chaos, the business meeting process is truly an opportunity to see how much you have grown and relinquished the need to control or resist perceived authority figures. These meetings can be a revelation. Business meetings cover elections, group policies, disbursements, liaison with host facility personnel, housekeeping, literature to be made available and matters of affiliation. They are usually informal, open to all and held at the conclusion of the regular group meetings.

Money Issues

Groups obtain operating expense money by taking a collection at each meeting. Any and all contributions are voluntary; there are *no* dues or fees for membership. Money is generally a minor issue for most groups because there are very few expenditures that a group needs to consider: rent for the facility, disbursement for nonaddictive refreshments and the purchase of literature (much of which is sold at cost).

Once current expenses and bills have been handled, the group may have a surplus and a question about how to spend it. I believe that money is only valuable when it is helping to carry the message. Consequently I suggest to most groups that they keep a prudent reserve (two or three months estimated expenses) and let go of all additional funds. Contributing to their national affiliate or to the local church or school that helped make the meeting possible all are creditable ways of using money to advance the spirit of ACoA.

Group funds need to be handled diligently and properly recorded each week. It helps to have a group treasurer who is precise, committed and concerned. If the proposed treasurer isn't able to meet these qualifications, perhaps the group should consider another individual for the task.

This task carries a clear-cut responsibility. Sometimes, because the group is nonprofit and the weekly collection is small, there is a tendency to be lax about records and deposits. Try to avoid this. Where substantial surpluses occur I urge the group to put the money to work. At least once every three months the treasurer needs to provide the group with an accounting.

Suggested Meeting Formats

Each group is an independent and autonomous body, and as such, it can select or develop any meeting format it considers will best fit its needs.

Standard Format

Some may opt for a standard format, which is comprised of a speaker who tells his or her story for 20 to 30 minutes followed by a one-hour open discussion. The discussion phase can involve either a directed (focused) topic such as "Handling feelings of abandonment," or it can be free-form with group members sharing whatever is on their minds.

The structure of the meeting is also optional. For a typical discussion meeting I find the following structure to be helpful:

1. Open the meeting with the Serenity Prayer.
2. Read a preamble (Statement of Purpose).
3. Ask each person to introduce himself or herself by first name only.
4. Reading of Laundry List and Solution.
5. Introduction of speaker, who qualifies for 20 to 30 minutes.
6. Secretary's break, collection.
7. Guided discussion with topic from ACoA 12 Steps or Laundry List and Solution.
8. Close the meeting with the Lord's Prayer.

Beginners' Meeting

Another meeting format is a one-hour meeting designated as a "Beginners' Meeting." In this format the chair usually conducts a 20-minute introductory session that focuses on elements and aspects of the program that can be helpful to newcomers to the program. Topics include the Laundry List, ACoA, the 12 Steps of recovery, the importance of attendance at meetings, sponsorship, developing friendships in the program, how meetings operate, cautions about confronting parents prematurely, literature that is recommended and the value of sharing and serving at meetings.

Beginners' meetings are structured along the same lines as the standard meetings, except that the chair generally does the sharing and the focus is exclusively on information for the newcomer. Some of the topics that I try to cover when I lead beginners' meetings include:

- A brief review of available ACoA literature for better knowledge and understanding.
- Attendance at a minimum of four to six meetings before making a decision about the program.
- Reach out and obtain telephone numbers of members, develop friendships and go out for a snack with members after the meeting.
- The role of a sponsor and the need for one.
- The importance of studying the ACoA 12 Steps of recovery and guidance from a sponsor.
- Newcomers are asked to sit in the front row, if possible, and to participate and share.
- Distribute "beginners' kits" to newcomers. These might include the Laundry List, a list of meetings and other explanatory information.

Affiliation

Some groups choose to maintain affiliation with a national organization. There are two, ACA and Al-Anon. A group that affiliates with Al-Anon must adhere to a distinct set of procedures and regulations. The Laundry List and Solution are not approved literature and cannot be read, distributed or discussed at meetings that choose to affiliate with Al-Anon. ACA does not have such restrictions. Many meetings claim that they function quite well as unaffiliated meetings. In most areas the time and meeting locale of unaffiliated meetings are listed along with those of affiliated groups.

Size of Meetings

As the ACoA movement grows and expands, more and more people are attending the meetings. This is wonderful; but problems can arise when the group size exceeds 20 or 25 members:

- Not everyone may get to share. ACoA was designed to be a forum where everyone who desires to can share. In larger meetings, members, particularly newcomers, can get lost in the shuffle.
- Not having an opportunity to share and be heard may be a painful reminder of what it was like as a child when we were not heard, not allowed to have a point of view or just plain ignored.
- The larger the meeting, the more intimidating and frightening it is for some. This can lead to a reluctance or fear of speaking.
- In a large meeting the newcomer may not be noticed or acknowledged. The sensitive or frightened newcomer may not gain a sense of belonging. I always urge groups to develop a standard procedure in the meeting to ensure that newcomers are acknowledged, given a "beginner's kit" and have an opportunity to ask questions. It's so easy for the lost child personality to blend into the woodwork and stay lost.

One suggestion I have for really large groups, say 30 or more members, is to hold two meetings back to back. Another way to handle overcrowding is to break up into smaller discussion groups right after the speaker qualifies. Discussion groups of eight to ten people enable everyone to share, especially those who find it difficult to share when there is a large audience. Over the years I have found that small discussion groups tend to produce a deeper, more personal sharing. The size of the audience tends to dictate the level of sharing for some members. Since one of the cornerstones of ACoA is personal sharing (revealing the family secrets and our own issues), a principal mission of any group should be to facilitate this sharing in every way possible.

Anonymity

AA, the original 12-Step recovery program, considers anonymity to be the foundation of its program. This concept is equally important to the ACoA recovery program. Some of the key aspects of our anonymity stance are as follows:

- Whatever we may hear shared at a meeting must be kept confidential. What we hear in the meeting rooms should stay in the meeting rooms. We must always respect the confidentiality of the members.
- A member should especially guard against ever revealing the names of ACoA members to nonmembers or the public at large. Each individual's affiliation with ACoA is a private and personal matter and we, as fellow members, must respect this right to privacy. Our sense of security and support require it.
- At the individual level a member may elect to reveal his or her own association with ACoA to another individual or group of nonmembers. Such action should be undertaken with caution as such disclosure may cause harm to an innocent relative or family member.
- At the public media level I urge discretion concerning revealing one's association with ACoA. Broad publicity, though well meant, may reflect negatively on parents and relatives. When it comes to public disclosure to the media it is best to look carefully at the content of the situation and the motives involved. Some have found it freeing to reveal the family secrets, while others have found that it increased family disharmony. On this issue each member would do best to seek the guidance of his or her Higher Power.

Starting A New ACoA Group

Fortunately the logistics of starting a new ACoA group are reasonably easy to grasp. Negotiation generally involves the arrangements regarding a meeting room. Most churches, hospitals, rehabilitation and therapy centers and some municipal build-ings often make space available for local community self-help organizations. They typically charge a small rental fee for use of a meeting room.

A second task when forming a new group will be to publicize it. Typically those starting it will visit other ACoA groups and inform the members of the new group's formation. Some new group officers also publicize the new meeting to mental health facilities, hospitals, church counselors, schools, rehabilitation organizations and individual therapists. A primary source is the national organization, if the group chooses to affiliate with one. Local HELP lines and community clearinghouse organizations also can be a way to expand knowledge of the group.

If you decide to start an independent group, the only tools you need are your knowledge of how 12-Step self-recovery meetings typically function and some basic literature such as the Laundry List, Solution and perhaps this book. If you decide to affiliate with Al-Anon or ACA, you should write or call the state (local) office or national headquarters for guidance.

Some Personal Stories Of ACoA Members

CHAPTER 12

Evelyn's Story

I was an only child. My father left my mother shortly after I was four years old, and I rarely saw him during my early years. I wanted him to settle down so I could leave my mother and go live with Dad. Well, it never worked out that way. He had no idea of what I was all about or what needs I had. He just couldn't be there for me.

When my father left us, my mother and I became a team — "You and me against the world," she once said. For a few years that's how we functioned, but by the time I was nine years old it became my mom against me. By then her drinking had become so bad that it was just tearing us apart.

My mother had been born and raised in Germany and came to this country in the late 1950s. She was rigid in her views, and highly controlling. She had very set ideas about how her daughter should act. My behavior was constantly being monitored and strictly enforced. In short, I was being smothered at an early age and I just hated it.

Mom and I lived in a tenement apartment in a big city. We never had much money, but she was a responsible worker who dutifully showed up for her work every day. We had very little social life. My mother knew very few people. As her alcohol-

117

ism progressed she spent most nights and weekends at home.
She isolated herself terribly.

My days were pretty unsupervised after I was nine years
old. I had one really close friendship with a schoolmate named
Debbie, who lived across the street. We became inseparable.
She was the only person I could really trust and confide
in. She and her family were always there. I could count on
them to help me whenever I was in trouble with Mom or
school officials.

I started my revolt against my mother by the time I turned
ten. I also began acting out at school, and between the ages of
ten and 19 my life was pure hell. Emotionally I was barely
getting by. My mother and I had arguments almost every
night. They were impossible battles filled with drunken
screaming and bitter accusations. All my mother's
disappointments were being heaped on me. Her frustration
with my behavior came out in many ways. Usually it was the
age-old criticism, "You can't do anything right. I can't count
on you for anything."

Well, it wasn't too long before I obliged her by trying to do
things my way instead of hers. A part of me desperately
wanted my mother's love and approval, but the rebellious brat
in me kept resisting her. On those rare occasions that I got a
good grade at school, my mother would discount it and focus
on all my poor grades. I just couldn't win.

As my resistance to her grew, her punishment escalated.
Verbal abuse was an everyday event. Somehow she thought
that physical beatings, spankings and random slaps in the face
would have a positive effect on me. In drunken rages she even
chased me around the apartment with a kitchen knife.

I remember thinking that I wasn't allowed anyone or
anything that might give me even a small chance of happiness.
I clung to Debbie and her family, and spent many nights in
their home when my mother "accidentally" locked me out of
our apartment.

My mom had no religion and didn't believe in any God, and
living with her could be quite dangerous. One drunken night
my mother gave me Lysol by accident instead of cough syrup.
Then she railed at me for her mistake. Everything was my
fault. According to her I was worthless, stupid and inadequate, and all of this required frequent punishment.

I acted tough and rebellious on the outside, but I was very shy and frightened much of the time. I wanted to be part of a loving and caring family, but knew it was impossible. The saddest part of those years is that my mother believed she was doing everything for me that was possible.

My escape came in the form of music. I studied opera singing and became very accomplished — so much so that at age twelve I was performing with a large local opera company. Unfortunately success took much practice, which became almost impossible as my mother would listen and ridicule me more and more with each successive drink. Finally I just gave it up — the pain and criticism and my low self-esteem all worked against me.

Another escape for me was sleep. As I grew into my teens I began going to bed earlier to avoid my mother's drunken ravings. I didn't always sleep well. A part of my mind was always alert to mother's stage of drunkenness and the possible threat it posed. Often she would charge drunkenly into my bedroom to accuse me or berate me. One night things got very bad. I sensed that something was very amiss. I got up to check and discovered that she had passed out — but had put on the gas jets in an attempt to kill herself, and probably me!

Through my teens we argued and screamed at each other daily. In many ways I was becoming just like her and it frightened me. At school I aligned myself with the rebels, the defiant and negative ones. Often I skipped class. I cared little for myself and less about school or a career. When I graduated from high school, I moved into my own small studio apartment, got a job and slowly learned how to take care of myself. I began to take some college courses and began what I thought was a new and safer life. I was wrong.

Thanks to Ma Bell, abuse was only a phone call away. It got so that Mom didn't even have to call me. I was very talented at beating myself up and being consumed by self-doubt. All those years of being told I was worthless and useless had caught up with me. The voices in my head were very powerful. I believed myself to be all those things my mother said about me. I wasn't safe and I wasn't free. I was feeling miserable and looked for ways to escape from myself. I seriously thought about moving to Europe. I looked desperately for a relationship

that would save me. I had no direction or understanding of
myself or what was happening to me. I felt lost and alone.

My best friend, Debbie, came to my rescue. She took me to
Al-Anon, Alateen and — luckily — to ACoA. While I identified
strongly with the members of ACoA, I felt that I could get
along without it. I stopped attending meetings for a while and
very quickly fell back into a miserable, desperate isolation. So,
without prompting from Debbie, I went back to ACoA with a
purpose, and was amazed at how quickly I began to change. It
was mostly surface change at first, but it was a start.

I began to feel that I was among friends, that I could trust
people at meetings. I was able to cry, shout and be angry. I let
all the pain come out of me. People accepted me. No one
blamed me. As I let the lid off all my terrible feelings, I began
to get better. Some days I thought those feelings were going
to kill me — and I was only 20 years old. When I heard another member tell a similar story to mine, I was moved to tears
with gratitude that I wasn't alone.

There were many days in my early recovery when I didn't
want to be in touch with my feelings. But the members
supported me and gave me the courage to move forward and
stay with the pain. It was finally learning all about growing
up, a process I missed in my alcoholic home. I learned how
to be my own father and mother.

After much effort and anger, I got to the point where I
could accept and forgive my mother. It wasn't easy, but I will
be forever grateful to ACoA, because my mother and I finally
got to say the things that needed to be said before her early
and untimely death at the age of 47.

Jenny's Story

Sometimes it's difficult for me to be clear about what really
happened in my home when I was growing up. I was one of
three girls. My father was a small-town lawyer and my
mother was a schoolteacher. My father was a liberal free
spirit, while my mother was a conservative, coldly disciplined
taskmaster.

Dad was fun-loving, congenial and the life of the party, but
he got to the point where he began to enjoy liquor more than
most other pleasures. By the time I was four or five he had

began to use alcohol on a daily basis. At first he seemed full of life and good cheer but, as time passed, he began to turn nasty and mean when he drank too much. Many nights I lay awake listening to my mother and father argue.

Mom was always angry about my father's drinking and she took every opportunity to badger and berate him about it. Eventually the arguments spilled over into the dinner meal. I remember getting knots in my stomach and being unable to eat. My little sisters (I was the oldest) would cry and whimper whenever an argument would erupt at dinner. By the time I was eight or nine years old, life began to get pretty miserable at home. It was about this time that my father's drinking really changed him.

One night when I was trying to concentrate on my homework, Mom was out and Dad was stumbling around. He asked me to get him something. Before I could get up and do it he slapped me with real force right in the face. It almost knocked me over. I ran out of the room crying and trembling. He yelled after me that I had better "Jump to it!" when he asked for something. I felt devastated and hurt. Over the summer months he slapped me a few more times and raged at all of us children.

I got so I didn't trust my dad anymore. I became wary, suspicious and began avoiding him. While all this was happening, my mother started to really put pressure on me to achieve and be "little Miss Perfect." It was as if the worse things got at home, the more my mother wanted us all to paint a portrait of family tranquility. It was made very clear to me that I was never to tell anyone about the family secret — my father's drinking. My mom used to complain bitterly, "It's a damned shame." And that's just what I felt — shame.

By the time I was 12 my mother started getting abusive to all of us. Dad stayed away from home a lot, as his practice was getting successful despite his drinking. He must have been a real manipulator with his clients. The county was growing and he was doing a lot of real estate law. One night I heard my mother accuse my father of having an affair with a local woman. I was mortified. Maybe I couldn't trust his moods but this was just plain abandonment.

He didn't care about any of us. After this incident I grew very distant and avoided him whenever I could. He recognized what I was doing and often made nasty remarks about it. He called me "Miss High and Mighty" and "Her Majesty the Snob."

Up until this point I had very mixed feelings about my father. On the one hand I wanted his affection and praise, and I tried to get it by being perfect. At the same time I was angry at him for what he was doing, his physical abuse of me and harsh criticism when he was drunk. I guess I both loved him and despised him and I felt rejected. Way at the bottom of my feelings were two issues: I didn't trust him and I felt rejected. And I was rebelling against my mother's overcontrolling ways. I was a pot that was ready to boil over.

When I was 14, I discovered boys and the pot did indeed boil over. I was so ready — just desperate for attention and affection, I used boys and men to escape from the mess at home. I just turned myself over to their care. I truly lost myself in them. My schooling suffered, my mom tried to restrict me more and I had vicious fights with her. She began accusing me of being "loose." It was true — but I denied it.

I had very few friends at school. I had trouble with friendships, I had trouble with teachers, I had trouble with boyfriends and I had trouble with my parents. I felt like I *was* trouble.

Even my little sisters began battling with me. Despite all this turmoil and family trouble, I wasn't drawn to drugs or alcohol. If anything I was very much against them. Oh, I did try pot and a few beers, but I was not tempted. I guess men had become my substance of choice. Toward the end of my senior year I got pregnant and eventually had an abortion. My parents were not very supportive and this incident became another mechanism that distanced me.

By now my folks had developed a stony, sterile way of living. They were going through the motions but there was no love left, just duty and obligation. There was even less communication. My mother was running a household to gain approval and recognition. It was all a "very proper" show and each of us had a part to play. I felt like such a phoney!

While I was at college, two important changes occurred in my life. I became very interested in doing well and did, in fact, graduate with honors. And I fell in love and married a medical student who became a pediatrician. My mother was very happy about these changes. Even my father gave me grudging approval for making a stable and sensible choice.

It may have been sensible but it sure wasn't perfect. I was very much into control and this pattern, along with my tendency to distrust and withhold affection and feelings, caused great problems. I wanted a mate who would fit my fairytale image — and that's just not reality.

I tended to be abusive and hysterical when very upset and this really hurt our relationship. As they say in ACoA, I was a composite of the dominant traits of my mother and father — so my husband really had his hands full.

Finally things got so tense that I entered therapy and began unearthing the family secrets. Eventually my therapist suggested that I attend some ACoA meetings, and I did.

The rest is history — and thank God, recovery.

Frank's Story

My childhood years were no picnic. Luckily for me, I had no way of knowing just how bad it was. I grew up in a blue-collar, working-class family. I was the youngest of two children. Both of my parents drank, but only my mother had difficulty with it.

By the time I was five years old, my mother had perfected a pretty miserable way of handling the stresses and strains in her life. She would simply get drunk and abandon us for about four days or so. There was never any warning or signal from her. She never told us what she was planning or when she was leaving, and she never apologized to any of us for her behavior. Evidently she had worked it out that it was her right to just walk out on us whenever she felt the urge.

She would usually slip out of the house late at night (my father worked nights) and creep or stumble back in four days later. She would disappear, on average, about once a month and maintained this pattern right up until she died in her early 50s. By the time that I was seven or eight years old, I had become accustomed to her binges. On the surface I seemed to adjust to her sickness in pretty much the same way that my sister and father had. All this abandonment took its toll, but somehow I had learned how to act as if my mother was fine, just a little eccentric.

Concealing my mother's shameful behavior was the most important task of the whole family. I can recall not bringing

my school chums into my house for fear that my mother
might return from a binge unexpectedly.

We had a pretty standard way of punishing my mother for
her actions. My father instructed me and my sister to give my
mother the "silent treatment" whenever she returned from a
binge. This wall of silence was to last for however long she
had been away. Thus, if she left us for four days, we would
punish her for four days. So at a very young age I was taught
that the way to deal with anger, disappointment and rejection
was to punish the person with silence — never, ever express
what you feel.

Unfortunately I was a frightened and needy little boy who
desperately wanted all the affection, concern and nurturing
love that I could get. I wasn't allowed to ask for any of these
things. I was forced to pretend that my mother didn't exist
though she might be only a few feet away and hurting as
badly as I was. Those years were incredibly painful for me, but
I didn't understand it then. Often I would lay awake at night,
waiting for my mother to start her journey out of the house. I
would slip out of bed and try to intercept her passage. There
were many nights that I intercepted her and pleaded with her.
My appeals never worked and she would be off on a drunken
visit to one of her girlfriends.

I blamed myself for her leaving. There was something that I
wasn't doing right, some way that I had failed her. I never did
figure out what it was. I became very sensitive to the possibility of people rejecting me and walking out on me. It didn't take
long for me to reason that I was unlovable and powerless.

It's not easy for me to describe my father. Rage, lightning
anger, overbearing control and intolerance were his principal
responses to life and a wayward drunken wife. In our family
my sister could do no wrong. She was very smart, beautiful
and the pride of my father. I was the one who could do no
right. I became the object of much of my father's wrath.
He was a firm believer in total obedience and frequent
punishment to break any habits that might lead to
individuality or independence. Beatings with a big leather
belt were frequent, as were vicious slaps to the face and head.
He was explosive, unpredictable and inconsistent. He was a
true bully and terrorized the entire family. For me he had
reserved a daily ration of criticism and derision. He taught me
to fear authority. He also taught me about self-loathing. I was

terminally dumb, clumsy and incompetent. And I had big ugly
ears. I can't recall that I ever sought advice from my father. I
was too frightened of him and his arbitrary reactions. His ridicule kept me from any attempt at a father-son relationship. So
early in life, I lost any chance to be connected to and cherished
by a father. He just didn't have the capacity for it.

Not long ago I saw the movie *A Field of Dreams*. It was all
about fathers and sons, the healthy kind. I couldn't stop crying
for 20 minutes at the end of the movie — something that I
never do. I guess that I'm still "experiencing out" some of that
deep hurt. I became very adept at avoiding my father and his
punishing ways. I also learned how to lie as a means of
protecting myself from beatings.

In so many unconscious ways my parents defined me. They
gave me my first portrait of myself and told me that it wasn't
very valuable to them or the world. I just wasn't worth much
consideration as a human being. I was never allowed to
confront, challenge or display anger. That kind of action
was reserved for my father only. My sister and I walked on
eggshells all the time lest we irritate my father or cause my
mother to start drinking. In those days I didn't know that
I couldn't cause the family illness and I couldn't control
or cure it.

When I qualify at an ACoA meeting, I often refer to the one
twisted benefit of the family sickness: Everything was very
predictable and certain. The roles were rigid and nothing
changed them as I grew up. You could count on my mother
getting drunk, disappearing for four days and returning to
isolate in silence for another four days. My father's rage was
just part of the daily fabric of family life. It was always just
beneath the surface or erupting. And, above all, there was fear
and self-hate everywhere. I sometimes wonder how I made it
out of my home with any kind of sanity. We children were
merely properties to be exploited and treated as the parents
saw fit. We had no rights, no opportunity to develop as
distinct individuals. We had no privileges or protection.

Throughout my teen years the family stayed stuck in this
sick and punishing dynamic. Nothing changed. I became the
family scapegoat but managed to escape into workaholism by
the time I was 14. Through work I gained some independence
and a little grudging admiration from my father. In high
school I became a people-pleaser. Other people's impressions

and opinions of me were far more important than mine. Like so many others who grew up in an alcoholic home, I became very defensive, hypervigilant and unfeeling. I did not see the world as a safe and secure place. People weren't to be trusted.

Armed with my father's distorted philosophy about life and people, I trotted off to the Marine Corps to see if I could prop up my low self-esteem with heroic deeds and courageous acts. Strange as it may seem, my four years with the Marines turned out to be very valuable to my getting free of my home. I shudder to think what it might have been like had I stayed enmeshed with my family. I had some good leadership qualities and some innate capabilities that took me through a war without a scratch. I advanced rapidly in rank and won an appointment to officer candidate school just as the war was ending. I elected to take a discharge and go to college.

In school I became fascinated with the idea of success and achievement. I wanted to be "somebody." I wasn't sure what, but I had this need for credentials and respect and wealth. Looking back I can see that it was one of my many efforts to compensate for very deep feelings of inadequacy. I was going to smother these old fears under a ton of credentials. So I raced through undergraduate school and won a complete fellowship for a Master's degree. I was building a somewhat tentative structure of self-worth, but the foundation was built on sand. There was still a frightened and helpless little kid in me who had not been dealt with. At this point in my life all of my actions were "other-directed." I had no real center. I was just tuning in to the prevailing signals of society: work hard, learn, achieve, acquire and look good.

By the time I was 30 it all began to come apart. I had blindly followed the "other" voices and didn't have a clue as to who I was or what I was about. I began feeling a sense of isolation, a feeling that I didn't belong anywhere. I also began questioning my talents and my direction. I was beginning to feel lost and helpless again. On the surface I was friendly and personable. I was a fairly capable businessman but I was intimidated by authority figures, had difficulty communicating with my subordinates and had trouble confronting people and telling them what my needs were. I expected people to automatically understand my hidden agenda. Overall I was more interested in form than in content. It was very important to "look good."

In my relationships I was shallow, inconsistent and overly sensitive. I didn't know how to communicate or challenge softly. Sometimes I was a real hammer in my dealings with people, I was also far too arrogant and unyielding, probably a carry over from my days as a drill instructor in the Marines. I had no notion of sharing and I needed to be in control of my environment and the people in it. I had great difficulty just letting events unfold.

Where romance was concerned, I never got beyond the primitive sexual stages. I didn't have any idea how to be with people emotionally. Now I see that for many years I was scared to death of intimacy. I didn't have the slightest idea what it meant to be vulnerable and open to someone. I had no empathy and no compassion. I was domineering and angry just like my father. And, sadly, I just kept repeating my patterns in one relationship after another. I was emotionally punishing to women. I used silence and abandonment or indifference as my major weapons. I was very much a composite of my parents' worst behavior patterns.

In my mid-30s I began to experience anxiety and panic, emotions that I had always kept stuffed. Behind this were all the feelings of inadequacy and worthlessness that I had somehow buried as a helpless little boy. Now my efforts at control were failing me and I was very frightened. I also made some bad decisions at work and found myself face to face with my own limited capabilities. I wanted maximum return with minimum vulnerability and life wasn't working out to my satisfaction.

As my anxiety grew — and it did so very quickly — I sought professional help. In therapy my long-hidden pain emerged. I felt terrible for months. Fortunately I had an enlightened therapist who suggested that I join a local ACoA self-help group. I was very hesitant about this and arrived at my first meeting full of defenses, suspicion and fear. But something happened that night. I still can't explain what it was. I think it was some kind of spiritual shift, some kind of surrender, whatever it was it worked.

Since that first meeting, my life has changed a great deal. I've learned to trust, be vulnerable, share and sit with all the painful early feelings. I've had to deal with all those early feelings of helplessness and inadequacy. I now have a pretty

solid understanding of who I am, and I really like who I am
and what I do.

Mary Lee's Story

My parents had me late in life. My sister was 16 years older
than I, and three brothers followed her closely in age. I was
the fifth child.

My entire family was actively alcoholic. Drinking was
permitted at our home even though it was prohibition years.
When I was six I saw a movie at school that showed a drunken
father being carried through the swinging bar-room doors and
the little son sobbing at the sight of his father. I told this story
to the family at dinner and was reprimanded unmercifully for
accusing my father of drunkenness. He was a successful
businessman who was active in community affairs. He was
also an inventor, designer and first violinist in the civic
orchestra. He was hardly ever at home. And when he did
come home drunk, his job was to discipline the errant child
with a cowhide whip. I spent these violent times under
the bed so I wouldn't hear the screams and cries.

My mother was never supportive of me. She always
introduced me as the reason she did not go to California. She
certainly did not nurture me. I spent my entire life trying to
please her and make her see me, but she never did. I did not
count as a family member. When she died at 89 years,
I felt relief.

I was disliked by all my siblings. With my birth, my sister
was no longer the only girl; my youngest brother was no
longer the baby. As the youngest, hated child, I was
persecuted, slapped by any member of the family, teased,
violated. I was sexually abused by a brother and mentally and
physically abused by them all.

I grew up a guilty human being, full of shame, self-hatred,
confusion, frustration, a child unloved, unwanted and helpless.
I was a lost child. I never understood the insane behavior of my
family. No one was there for me. I was just not seen or heard.

These years of survival were years of emotional, spiritual
and physical deprivation. I did not know love. I learned not to
feel, not to talk and not to trust. I lived watching my elders'
lives unfold — marriages and grandchildren.

Yet there was one happy note: music. I taught myself to play piano and to write music. My theme was always death and heaven. Annie, the maid, taught me hymns, and as I played them, we sang together in harmony. These were my first prayers to God and I thank Annie for these precious moments.

When I was 11 years old, I was sent to a Catholic girl's academy far away. I traveled to school alone in the dark and returned home alone in the dark, so I was not permitted time to learn the joys of healthy sports or just fun. Even at this early age I felt I did not belong anywhere.

My first noticeable anxiety attacks occurred in this school. These I suffered for 48 years, relieved only by my use of alcohol.

When my father denied me transfer to a fine school nearby, I never asked anything of my father again, nor did I ever speak to him again. He cried at my graduation but, I refused to embrace him.

I attended a coed university. I was a good student, I made friends, I was accepted by the sorority of my choice and I was photographed as one of the best new freshmen women. I was in heaven. I was seen and heard at last.

Then my father died. My family sent me a telegram — no phone call, just a telegram.

I attended the funeral. A few days later the family fighting and drinking decided my college future. I could return.

But college was not the same for me. That spark of light and hope simply died.

I could not cope with the demands of school, so I became a success as a party girl. I could drink quite a bit and sing any college song. I was popular and I felt grown up at last.

I married and had two children. I marvel at how they grew up into the sensible human beings that they are today, for I was not a good mother.

In the following years I wore many hats. I continued to please the whole world. I was a mother, housewife, active corporate secretary, business entertainer, traveler, boatswoman, airplane co-pilot.

I spent all my vacations working on my boat. I took 35 or more trips, crossing the Gulf Stream and sailing to islands in the Caribbean. It was dangerous, frightening. My airplane travel took me through Central and South America through drug-infested territory and flea-infested lodgings. I could not refuse to go on these trips. I was trapped by my own refusal to say no. I feared abandonment, rejection, loneliness. I did not know who I was.

When I finally hit an alcoholic bottom, I was at home and alone. The psychiatrist assured me that I was an alcoholic. I thanked him profusely. At last I was something.

But nothing changed for me. I still believed that some person, place or thing or situation would make me happy.

I was a dry alcoholic. I stuffed my feelings more and more. I obliterated pain from my mind and continued to please everyone. I gave away more and more of my power.

I did not find fulfillment, for I was still alone and lonely. I was forever on the move and I ceased feeling altogether. But I kept hearing the words, "I want you for something." I heard them over and over and I knew God called me.

Home at last, I began therapy. It was vital for me to remain in one place and this decision entailed taking many risks. I was afraid of abandonment, rejection, loneliness, threats of financial insecurity, yet I suffered all this anyway. My needs were not met and I felt unloved and unwanted as a human being.

I read every self-help book offered to me; books I bought and books on the library shelf. I became fascinated with the study of me. I entered church programs. I became a volunteer at the hospital. I worked in detox, studied and worked the hospice program. I returned to college and earned 16 credits. I became a realtor and served as a trustee on the board of an alcoholic treatment center.

I made some new friends and I found ACoA. I began to reach out, listen and share. I identified with the stories of deprivation and emotional suffering. I liked the Problem Solution. I loved the program and I had a support group.

I began to uncover the stifled and hidden resentments, angers and fears of my childhood. I tried verbal confrontations with my family to share my feelings, but they chose not to see me or hear me. I wrote each one a letter telling them how it was for me. What's to lose, I thought, I never knew them anyway. Two years later, my brother responded as best he could and a few years later I attended his funeral joyous, happy and free, for I placed him with my deceased family in heaven.

Emotionally I was 19 years old when I began this therapy. I have journeyed through a grieving process. I now feel, hope. I felt I was an adult learning coping skills. I felt I climbed many rungs of Maslow's ladder of self-fulfillment.

But it was not true. I was not at rest. Quite unexpectedly, I hit a devastating new emotional bottom. Without warning and seeming provocation, I sobbed. My entire body shook. My entire life passed before me. I saw and felt every abuse, violation, deprivation that had been inflicted on me. Once again I hated myself for accepting this lifetime of abuse because I feared abandonment, rejection, loneliness.

I was experiencing a spiritual rebirth. I accepted the necessary grieving process and I surrendered my entire will to God.

Two days later I entered a treatment center, full of enormous courage and humility, beginning yet another journey. Life is a series of journeys, not a goal. But now I felt assurance, self-confidence that I was on the right path at last. God was now with me, and I walked into this treatment with honesty, openness and willingness. My feelings about doing this were positive.

I became like a blotter, a sponge. I soaked up all that I saw, heard and felt. I was again finding the real me.

And one marvelous day in Tony A's meditation class I got in touch with my inner child, a sad and lonely child. I picked her up, hugged her and sobbed with my child. A woman comforted me. I felt her compassion transfer itself to me. More meditations brought my child to me again. I saw my child, red-cheeked, glowing, smiling, dressed in night clothes, clutching a toy, pirouette around the living room, throw kisses to all and run laughing up the stairs.

I qualify as a co-dependent. I had low self-esteem, emotional deprivation, hated myself, came from a dysfunctional home, and was always looking outside myself for happiness. I was a people-pleaser with feelings of isolation, depression and fears.

I received the tools I need in order to become a healthy person. I'm changing a lifetime of old behavior and attitudes.

Everything finally seemed to come together for me. I have definition. I am an ACoA, an alcoholic and a co-dependent. I feel a new excitement and my priorities are clear.

Appendix

Resources

Adult Children of Alcoholics
6381 Hollywood Boulevard, Suite #685
Hollywood, CA 90028
213-464-4423

Al-Anon/Alateen Family Group Headquarters, Inc.
P.O. Box 862, Midtown Station
New York, NY 10018-0862
212-302-7240

Alcoholics Anonymous (AA)
P.O. Box 459, Grand Central Station
New York, NY 10163-1100
212-686-1100

Cocaine Anonymous
World Service Office
(213) 559-5833

Coc-Anon
World Service Office
(818) 377-4317

Co-dependents Anonymous
P.O. Box 5508
Glendale, AZ 85312-5508
(602) 944-0141

Debtors Anonymous
General Service Board
P.O. Box 20322
New York, NY 10025-9992

Families Anonymous
P.O. Box 344
Torrance, CA 90501

Gamanon
P.O. Box 967
Radio City Station
New York, NY 10019

Gamblers Anonymous
P.O. Box 17173
Los Angeles, CA 90017

Incest Survivors Anonymous
P.O. Box 5613
Long Beach, CA 90805

Narcotics Anonymous
P.O. Box 9999
Van Nuys, CA 91409

Nar-Anon Family Groups
350 5th St., Ste. 207
San Pedro, CA 90731

National Association for Children of Alcoholics
31706 Pacific Coast Hwy.
South Laguna Beach, CA 92677

Overeaters Anonymous
4025 Spencer St., Ste. 203
Torrance, CA 90503

Parents Anonymous
National Office
6733 Sepulveda Boulevard
Los Angeles, CA 90045

Rutgers Center of Alcohol Studies
P.O. Box 969
Piscataway, NJ 08854
201-932-2190

Survivors Network
18653 Ventura Boulevard, #143
Tarzana, CA 91356

Suggested Reading

Black, Claudia. **It Will Never Happen To Me.** Denver, M.A.C., 1981.

Castine, Jacqueline. **Recovery From Rescuing.** Deerfield Beach, FL: Health Communications, 1989.

A Course In Miracles. Tiburon, CA: Foundation For Inner Peace, 1976.

Earll, Robert. **I Got Tired Of Pretending.** Tucson: Stem, 1983.

Fishel, Ruth. **The Journey Within: A Spiritual Path To Recovery.** Pompano Beach, FL: Health Communications, 1987.

Progoff, Ira. **The Practice of Process Meditation.** New York: Dialogue House, 1980.

Wegscheider-Cruse, Sharon. **Choicemaking.** Pompano Beach, FL: Health Communications, 1985.

Whitfield, Charles. **Healing The Child Within.** Pompano Beach, FL: Health Communications, 1987.

Wholey, Denis. **Becoming Your Own Parent.** New York: Doubleday, 1986.

Wills-Brandon, Carla. **Learning To Say No: Establishing Healthy Boundaries.** Deerfield Beach, FL: Health Communications, 1990.

Woititz, Janet Geringer. **Adult Children of Alcoholics.** Pompano Beach, FL: Health Communications, 1983.

Wolter, Dwight Lee. **Forgiving Our Parents.** Minneapolis: Comp-Care, 1988.

New Books . . .
from Health Communications

ALTERNATIVE PATHWAYS TO HEALING: The Recovery Medicine Wheel
Kip Coggins, MSW
This book with its unique approach to recovery explains the concept of the medicine wheel — and how you can learn to live in harmony with yourself, with others and with the earth.
ISBN 1-55874-089-9 $7.95

UNDERSTANDING CO-DEPENDENCY
Sharon Wegscheider-Cruse, M.A., and Joseph R. Cruse, M.D.
The authors give us a basic understanding of co-dependency that everyone can use — what it is, how it happens, who is affected by it and what can be done for them.
ISBN 1-55874-077-5 $7.95

THE OTHER SIDE OF THE FAMILY:
A Book For Recovery From Abuse, Incest And Neglect
Ellen Ratner, Ed.M.
This workbook addresses the issues of the survivor — self-esteem, feelings. defenses, grieving, relationships and sexuality — and goes beyond to help them through the healing process.
ISBN 1-55874-110-0 $13.95

OVERCOMING PERFECTIONISM:
The Key To A Balanced Recovery
Ann W. Smith, M.S.
This book offers practical hints, together with a few lighthearted ones, as a guide toward learning to "live in the middle." It invites you to let go of your superhuman syndrome and find a balanced recovery.
ISBN 1-55874-111-9 $8.95

LEARNING TO SAY NO:
Establishing Healthy Boundaries
Carla Wills-Brandon, M.A.
If you grew up in a dysfunctional family, establishing boundaries is a difficult and risky decision. Where do you draw the line? Learn to recognize yourself as an individual who has the power to say no.
ISBN 1-55874-087-2 $8.95

SUBSCRIBE TO THE MAGAZINE DEVOTED TO ADULT CHILDREN

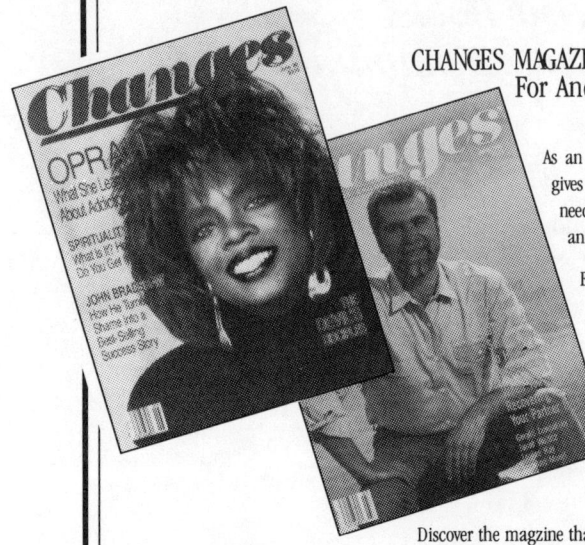

CHANGES MAGAZINE
For And About Adult Children

As an Adult Child, Changes Magazine gives you the vital self-healing tools you need to understand your inner child and recover from a traumatic past.

Each copy of Changes brings you new information on today's recovery concerns like self-esteem, intimacy, relationships and self-parenting. Plus you'll receive news on ACoA issues, support groups, recovery techniques, and 12-Step programs.

Discover the magzine that's helping Adult Children across the United States to develop genuine inner peace and personal satisfaction.

TRY **CHANGES** RISK FREE WITH OUR MONEY-BACK GUARANTEE.
JUST RETURN THE COUPON BELOW OR CALL TOLL-FREE 1-800-851-9100.

Yes, please begin my subscription to **Changes Magazine**. If I'm unsatisfied I can cancel my subscription within 30 days after I receive my first issue and promptly receive a full refund. After 30 days, I'm guaranteed a full refund on all unmailed issues.

Name _____
(please print)

Address _____ Apt. _____

City _____ State _____ Zip_____

Payment: ___ 1 Year (6 Issues) $18.00   ___ 2 Years (12 Issues) $34.00
___ Check (Payable to **The U.S. Journal**)   ___ Mastercard   ___ Visa
Acct. No. _____

Exp. Date _____ Signature _____
                                                    Response Code HDCHG1

SEND TO: The U.S. Journal Inc./Subscriptions
           3201 SW 15th St.
           Deerfield Beach, FL 33442-8190